Be a Survivor™

Colorectal Cancer Treatment Guide

Second Edition

VLADIMIR LANGE, MD

Be a Survivor™
Colorectal Cancer Treatment Guide, Second Edition

Vladimir Lange, M.D.

© Copyright 2006, 2009, 2011 by Lange Productions.
All rights reserved.
No part of this book may be reproduced in any manner without
written permission. For information contact Lange Productions,
7661 Curson Terrace; Los Angeles, CA 90046. 1-888-LANGE-88

ISBN 978-0-9819489-4-2

Second Printing, 2nd Edition, April 2014

A CIP record for this book is available from the Library of Congress.

Printed in the United States of America

Be a Survivor™
Colorectal Cancer Treatment Guide
Second Edition

VLADIMIR LANGE, MD

Lange
PRODUCTIONS

LOS ANGELES

TABLE OF CONTENTS

EXPERT CONTRIBUTORS FOR
BE A SURVIVOR - COLORECTAL CANCER TREATMENT GUIDE,
SECOND EDITION

THE UNIVERSITY OF CALIFORNIA, IRVINE HEALTHCARE
TEAM OF CONSULTANTS

Michael J. Stamos, MD

Joseph C. Carmichael, MD
Steven D. Mills, MD
Alessio Pigazzi, MD
Lari Wenzel, PhD
Jason A. Zell, DO

ADDITIONAL CONTENT CONTRIBUTION
Andrew Spiegel, CEO Colon Cancer Alliance

**The first edition of this book was developed
with the invaluable assistance of**

Robert W. Beart, MD, Yolee Casagrande, RN
Syma Iqbal, MD, Heinz-Josef Lenz, MD
Sandra A. Masson, RN, BSN, George Moro, MD
Stephen Shibata, MD, and Judith L. Trudel, MD

ACKNOWLEDGMENTS

No single author can do justice to a topic as complex as colorectal cancer. It is the guidance, support and expertise of my many knowledgeable colleagues that make this book the balanced, informative and accurate tool that will help you and your loved ones deal with your disease.

I wish to express my sincere gratitude to colleagues who supported the creation of the first edition of this book. Among them, my classmate Robert Beart, MD and my friend Yolee Casagrande, RN deserve special thanks.

This second edition was made possible by a new team of colleagues, based at University of California, Irvine Healthcare, and spearheaded by Michael Stamos, MD. He, and the experts he assembled, were instrumental in ensuring that the book reflects the best of what has recently become available in colorectal cancer management.

All of us who worked on this book want to thank the patients—the ones from whom we learn so much and the ones who contribute to research studies that allow us to advance the treatment and understanding of the disease. This book is for you, and for those who will follow in your footsteps to recovery.

INTRODUCTION

Being told that you have cancer is a trying experience. Being told that you have cancer of the colon or rectum may be particularly frightening, because colorectal cancer has been the topic of many recent news publications and broadcasts. If you try to apply the information you gleaned from the media to your particular case, you may be overwhelmed and confused.

I am no stranger to confusion. Many years ago my wife was diagnosed with breast cancer. Even though both of us are physicians, we understood little, and remembered even less, of the torrent of information that was thrown at us during our initial meeting with the doctors. It was weeks before we were able to unravel all the details, and begin deciding on a course of treatment.

That confusion lead me to write *Be a Survivor – Your Guide to Breast Cancer Treatment*. Like this book, it is a simple, clear and balanced presentation of the facts, designed to complement the information you receive from your physicians. The book is now it its fifth edition, and on the "must read" list of most breast cancer organizations. Since its publication, not a week has gone by that I haven't received comments such "Great explanation of a very complex subject...," "Best ever...," "My constant companion..." These comments, and the desire to make the journey easier for others, spurred me to create *Be a Survivor – Colorectal Cancer Treatment Guide*. It is an equally simple and effective guide to an equally challenging disease.

To make this book as balanced and objective as possible, I worked closely with a select group of top medical experts in all fields related to colorectal cancer. Thanks to this multi-specialty approach, the information presented here reflects a broad scope of expertise, rather than a single specialist's point of view.

How to Use This Book

I organized the book in a way that mirrors your path through treatment and recovery. It starts with suggestions on how to cope with the feelings you might experience after you learn that you have colorectal cancer, and a few tips on how to assemble a network of skilled healthcare providers to ensure that you get the best care possible. Think of it as building a safety net.

The rest of the book presents detailed descriptions of the various treatments you may encounter: surgery, radiation, chemotherapy and complementary medicine. Not all of them will be relevant to your case, but it is good to have a bird's eye view of the topic.

One of the chapters is written for your partner—husband, wife, or special man or woman in your life. This chapter will help her or him to be the best supporter for you, while dealing with her or his own needs during this time.

Each chapter includes lists of questions that you might want to address to your healthcare professionals. For your convenience, these questions are repeated at the end of the book. Take these sheets with you on office visits, to help you communicate more effectively with your physicians and nurses.

Since colon cancer and rectal cancer share many features, they are often referred to as "colorectal cancer." In some sections of this book, the two conditions are discussed together, in others separately to reflect ways in which treatments differ.

Use this book as a guide to help you understand all aspects of your treatment and recovery, and become an active member of your medical team. I, and the many skilled and dedicated healthcare professionals who worked with me on this book, wish you a speedy recovery.

CHAPTER 1

FACING COLORECTAL CANCER

When your learned that you have colorectal cancer, you were probably flooded with a host of emotions—fear, anger, confusion. You may have felt crushed—or in complete denial. You probably didn't remember any of the information, and you have no idea how to begin dealing with your situation. This is perfectly normal.

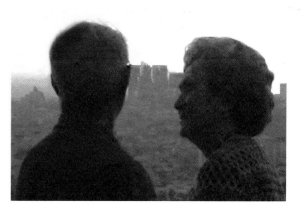

First of all, realize that a diagnosis of cancer is not a death sentence. A lot of progress has been made in the field, and survival rates today are higher than ever before.

Your first task is to decide that you will do everything you can to be successful in your battle against this cancer. This positive attitude will be your best ally throughout treatment and recovery. So, where to begin? Here are the initial steps you need to take to get control of the situation:

- Acknowledge your feelings, realize that they are normal, but don't let them affect your judgement.

- Assemble a network of healthcare professionals, friends and peers to help you deal with the situation.

- Contact a patient advocacy group, such as the Colon Cancer Alliance, to connect with other cancer survivors.

- Learn all you can about the disease and the different treatment options.

- Most importantly, become an active participant in your treatment and recovery.

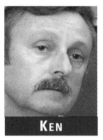

KEN

To begin with, the diagnosis of cancer was totally devastating. Then to be told that I'd have to have a hole in my stomach and wear a bag was a one-two knockout punch that was unbearable. I just broke down and cried, I think for the first time in my life.

UNDERSTANDING YOUR FEELINGS

The first few weeks after your diagnosis may be the hardest to handle. You may spend hours dwelling on questions such as "Why me?" or "Will the cancer kill me?" Or you might find yourself feeling "blue" and depressed to the point of not caring about the outcome of your disease. You might snap in anger at friends or loved ones.

This confusing roller coaster is natural. Don't be too hard on yourself if your emotions slip out of your control every once in a while. At a time like this, no one will expect you to be in perfect balance all the time.

The best approach is to find someone you can talk to about what you are experiencing. This should be a mature, well-adjusted person who can listen without passing judgment. Very close friends or family members may not be the best choice, because they can be too involved in the situation to remain objective.

Ask your doctor, nurse, or social worker for a referral for professional counseling, or to a local support group of cancer survivors who meet regularly, or are present online, to offer mutual support.

Psychiatrists, psychologists, and social workers can be very helpful with problems such as depression, panic attacks, feelings of isolation, and other issues that concern you.

SHARING THE NEWS

Communicating With Your Partner

Try to remember that your spouse or partner probably will be affected by your diagnosis as much as you. It is best to involve her or him as soon as possible, so the two of you can find strength in each other, and learn from the beginning how you can work as a team.

Both of you should feel free to discuss concerns with each other, as well as with your doctor, nurse, or other counselor who can give you the information and the reassurance you need.

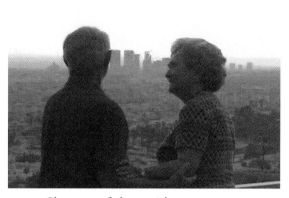

Share your feelings with your spouse

In some ways the spouse's or partner's challenge may be particularly difficult because he or she will have to manage his or her own emotions, and at the same time shoulder the task of being your supporter, helper, and sounding board.

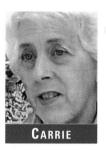

CARRIE

Sometimes it was hard to understand what the doctors said. But my husband…he would explain it to me. He is so organized. It was good to have him along.

Telling Your Family

The people who are close to you also will be affected by your news. They too may need to be angry, cry, and express their emotions. It's a natural part of adjusting to your diagnosis. It will help both you and them to talk openly about each other's feelings. Open communication from the start will go a long way toward strengthening the bonds with your loved ones, and securing the support you'll need.

Dealing with Friends and Others

Friends can be an excellent source of help and support, particularly if you keep them informed, and help them help you.

Most will want to help, but may be unsure of how to go about it, and will be waiting for clues from you about where to begin. Make specific requests for simple things. Ask them to run an errand, prepare a meal, come for a visit. These small acts bring friends back into contact and help them feel useful and needed.

Bear in mind that people who don't have experience dealing with cancer may have no idea what is acceptable. "Isn't it too personal to ask about her colostomy?" or "Should I pretend nothing happened?" or "How do I discuss his fears with him, without making things worse?" Help them by being the first to bring up whatever subject you want to discuss.

SUGGESTIONS FOR FRIENDS WHO WANT TO HELP

- Stop by and bring a newspaper
- Bring the mail or other materials from the office
- Help redecorate a room
- Organize a getaway weekend for both of you
- Drop by and watch a favorite TV program
- Drive you to a chemotherapy session
- Invite your whole family out for a meal

ASSEMBLING YOUR SUPPORT NETWORK

One of your first steps after you hear your diagnosis should be to establish a network of people who can help you. This network will include your loved ones, your peer support groups, and of course a solid team of health-care professionals.

Friends and Family

Your loved ones will provide the emotional support and closeness you need, and help you sort out facts and fears.

Try to select one person—your spouse, partner, or best friend—who will accompany you when you meet with your doctors, or go to your treatments. This companion can help you ask questions, remember information, or write down instructions.

He or she can become the center of your support network, acting as your sounding board, helping you to evaluate information and to make decisions, coordinating support from friends and family, and at times shielding you from excessive attention.

Support Groups

Consider joining a support group. Support groups are groups of people who meet regularly, under the guidance of a trained facilitator, to discuss the participants' concerns. Some groups exist as online support communities.

Some groups meet only a few times; others are long-term, enabling members to work through problems. Some are composed of people with the same disease. Others are selected by age or background. Some are just for patients; others include family or other special people.

Support groups give you a chance to openly discuss your thoughts with others who are going through the same experience. Many hospitals consider some form of group counseling to be a necessary part of the standard treatment.

Visit the support group a couple of times before joining, so you can be sure that the peer mix meets your needs and expectations.

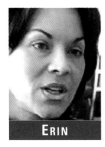

ERIN

Get into a support group both for you and your spouse. That is the best way to deal with the unknown. Surround yourself with people who have been there before.

YOUR HEALTHCARE TEAM

Cancer is a complicated disease and no single physician can be an expert in all aspects of the treatment.

Developing a treatment plan is a complex task that will involve a number of healthcare professionals — a whole team of experts — who will give you their advices and recommendations.

On the next page you will see, in alphabetical order, a list of most of the specialists who may be involved in your treatment. More than likely, there may be others.

Most facilities have teams of experts, called *multidisciplinary teams.* If your hospital doesn't, the National Cancer Institute, the Colon Cancer Alliance, or the American Cancer Society have resources to help you find healthcare professionals to add to your team.

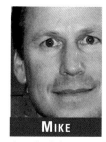

MIKE

As a firefighter, you feel that you are always in control. With a diagnosis of cancer, control was taken away - and suddenly I was treading very scary waters. It took a long time to regain my confidence.

Many hospitals have a *nurse navigator* who will guide you throughout the treatment and recovery process.

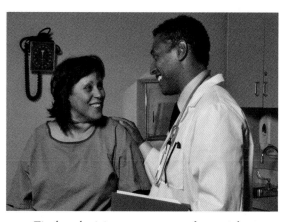

Find a physician you can get along with

Your satisfaction with your care, and the success of your treatment depend on finding healthcare professionals with whom you can get along, and who are willing and able to listen to your concerns. When selecting a surgeon, skill is an important factor. Feel free to question the surgeon about the number of procedures she or he had performed, and the success rate. A competent, confident professional will understand that your are concerned about your health, and will not take offense at your questions.

**QUESTIONS TO ASK
YOUR DOCTOR:**

- **Can I bring a member of my family, or a friend, to talk to you directly?**

- **What should I tell my loved ones about my condition?**

- **Can you refer me to a counselor or to a support group specializing in colorectal cancer?**

QUESTIONS TO ASK
YOUR DOCTOR:

• Tell me about
your experience
in dealing with
colorectal can-
cer.

• Could you give
me the names of
specialists you
think I should
see?

• How about
another set of
names so I can
choose the spe-
cialist(s) I like
best?

Members of your healthcare team

Anesthesiologist: Administers drugs or gasses that put you to sleep before surgery, and participates in pain control after surgery.

Clinical Nurse Specialist: A nurse with training or knowledge in a specific
area, such as post-operative care, chemotherapy, or radiation therapy.

Colorectal Surgeon: A surgeon with extensive additional training to become
a sub-specialist in colorectal surgery.

Enterostomal Therapist: A nurse or other health professional who teaches
patients how to live with, and care for ostomies and colostomy apparatus.

Gastroenterologist: A doctor who specializes in diagnosing and treating conditions affecting the digestive (gastrointestinal) tract.

Medical Oncologist: A doctor who administers anti-cancer drugs.

Nurse Navigator: A specially trained nurse who will be your guide during the
treatment process, and help you overcome obstacles with education and support.

Pathologist: A doctor who examines the tissue removed during a biopsy, and
issues a report to help your doctor choose the most effective treatment.

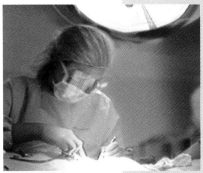

Pharmacist: A doctor of pharmacy who prepares and dispenses
prescribed medications.

Radiation Oncologist: A physician specially trained in using
high energy x-rays for treatment.

Radiation Therapy Technologist: A technologist who works
under the direction of the radiation oncologist to administer
radiation treatment.

Social Worker: A trained professional who can deal with social
and economic aspects of treatment, such as helping find a support group or
solving an insurance issue.

Surgeon: A doctor who performs a variety of general surgical procedures.

GETTING A SECOND OPINION

Selecting a treatment for your cancer is probably the most important issue you will ever face. For your own peace of mind, now and in the future, you may consider getting a "second opinion"—an evaluation of your case from another physician. Some patients are reluctant to do this, fearing that they may hurt the current doctor's feelings. Remember, it is your body. You are entitled to evaluate all your options, and no competent healthcare provider will object to your seeking another viewpoint.

Changing Doctors

Sometimes you may find that you are not getting along with one of the physicians treating you. The physician may seem abrupt, aloof, and uncaring, or fails to convince you of his or her competence. If this creates a barrier, let the physician know you wish to see someone else. The physician is probably as aware as you that a relationship based on trust and open communication has not been established, and will be happy to transfer your records to another practitioner.

To obtain a referral to a new physician, you may want to contact a reputable medical center or a local patient advocacy group, such as the Colon Cancer Alliance, or the American Cancer Society. Check the Reference section at the end of this book for other suggestions.

You should feel free to look for other physicians, but not if you are just shopping for a doctor who will promise a cure, or guarantee to relieve all your fears.

GATHERING INFORMATION

The more you know, the more active you can be in your own care. Becoming well informed about your cancer and about your options is one of the most important steps you can take at this stage. A firm grasp of the facts will give you a sense of comfort and control.

Your main source of information will be the professionals caring for you. Don't hesitate to ask any question, no matter how simple it may seem.

QUESTIONS TO ASK
YOUR DOCTOR:

- Do you, or your clinic or hospital, have a resource center? A library?

- Can you refer me to colorectal cancer groups or organizations in this area?

- Where can I find more information about colorectal cancer?

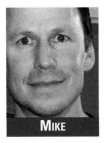

MIKE

Finding the best team of doctors to suit our needs was reassuring beyond belief. We walked out of the appointment full of hope. And hope is what you need to regain control, you know.

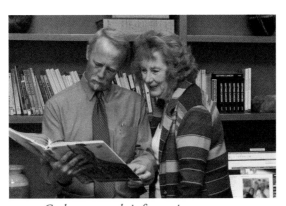

Gather as much information as you can

Ask your support person to accompany you to the medical appointments. That person will help you take notes, tape record what was said, or ask additional questions.

Make lists of topics you want to discuss, so that nothing is overlooked.

Use the tear sheets with suggested questions that are included at the end of this book as a guide for possible topics of discussion with your healthcare providers.

A lot of information—and, sadly, misinformation—is readily available on the internet. Be sure that the site you are consulting is managed by a reputable organization, and does not represent some individual's bias. If you have questions or concerns about any information you come across, let a member of your healthcare team know that you wish to discuss the information at your next appointment. Together you can evaluate what you read, and decide whether it is applicable to you.

On a regional or national level, there are several organizations that can be valuable sources of information. They can be found in the Resources section at the end of the book. The specialists at these organizations, many of whom are colorectal cancer survivors themselves, can answer many general questions about cancer, or send you written materials and information.

PLANNING YOUR TREATMENT

Planning your treatment should involve the entire team of specialists who consulted on your case, as well as your spouse, partner or your loved ones.

As your case progresses, your team of healthcare professionals will review the information available, and discuss your case with you and among themselves. You'll probably meet with various team members several

QUESTIONS TO ASK
YOUR DOCTOR:

• **Can you give me the name of a colorectal cancer expert who can give me a second opinion?**

• **Could you forward my chart, test results, and my biopsy slides to the doctor who is going to give me a second opinion?**

14

times, while they develop a recommendation for a course of treatment that's best suited to your case.

The key thing to remember is that it is you who will make the final decision, and all the members of the team need to respect it. That's why it is so important for you to learn all you can about your disease. The more information you can gather before you begin treatment, the better you will feel about your decision, and the more active role you'll be able to take.

Don't worry if you feel confused by the new words and concepts that you will come across. Most people do find them confusing at first. In the following days and weeks, as you explore this book, talk with your healthcare professionals, and gather additional information, you will become much more comfortable with the knowledge you need, and you will be able to make informed decisions.

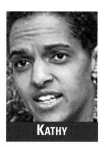

KATHY

They took out a bunch of lymph nodes, but I didn't get the pathology report right away. So that is when paranoia started to set in. "What are they not telling me?"

NOTES

CHAPTER 2

COLORECTAL CANCER BASICS

Before we discuss the treatment of colorectal cancer, let's first review a few points of anatomy. Some of the terms, like "lymph nodes" and "anal sphincter" may be unfamiliar to you, but they will help you understand the concepts better.

ANATOMY OF THE BOWEL

The main portion of our digestive tract is a tube that starts at the mouth, and includes the esophagus, stomach, small intestine and large intestine (also called colon), and ends with the rectum and anus.

As food travels down the digestive canal, it is processed by various specialized chemicals, called enzymes, into small particles. Along the way, these particles are gradually absorbed into the blood stream, to be distributed throughout the body and serve as a source of energy.

By the time the digested mixture gets down to the last part of the bowel, the colon, it is mostly waste—also called *stool* or *feces*. The colon absorbs any excess water from the stool, making it firm.

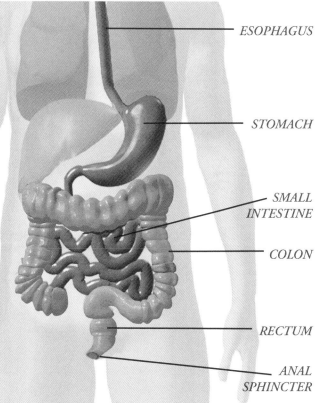

ESOPHAGUS

STOMACH

SMALL INTESTINE

COLON

RECTUM

ANAL SPHINCTER

The large intestine, the last part of the alimentary canal, consists of several parts. The *colon* itself, a muscular tube about five to six feet long, is made up of several parts: the *ascending, transverse,* and *descending* colon, which lie folded in your abdomen, and the *sigmoid* colon, which is mostly in the pelvis. The main function of the colon is to absorb as much moisture from the products of digestion, to create well-formed stools.

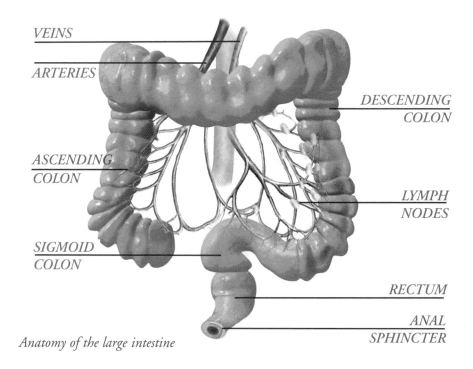

VEINS

ARTERIES

DESCENDING
COLON

ASCENDING
COLON

LYMPH
NODES

SIGMOID
COLON

RECTUM

ANAL
SPHINCTER

Anatomy of the large intestine

The last eight or ten inches of the digestive tract, the *rectum*, lies deep inside the pelvis. The rectum is the reservoir where stool is held prior to defecation. The rectum ends at the *anus*—the opening to the outside of the body. A circular band of muscles, called the *anal sphincter* surrounds the anus to keep it closed, so that stool does not leak out.

The wall of the large intestine is composed of multiple layers. The inner layer is called the *mucosa*. It contains cells that help absorb the digested food, and help keep bacteria out of the blood stream. These cells reproduce and die very rapidly—renewing the lining of the colon approximately every six days. Colorectal cancer originates from cells in this layer.

Arteries and veins carry blood to and from the intestine, supplying it with oxygen, and collecting nutrients to be used by the body. This network of blood vessels fans out in an apron-shaped layer called the *mesentery*.

The human body has an ability to compensate for the loss of part, or even most, of the colon without significant loss of efficiency.

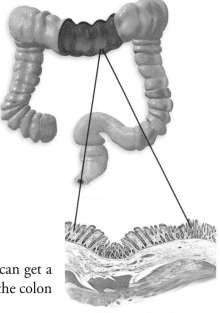

An important concept to understand is the *lymphatic system*. Lymph is the fluid that leaks out of the blood vessels and accumulates between cells. Lymph ducts collect this fluid and return it to the main circulation. Along the way, lymphatic fluid is filtered through small bean-shaped structures called *lymph nodes*, which trap debris such as bacteria, or escaped cancer cells. You may think of the lymphatic system as a network of sewer lines, although it also plays an important role in your immune defense system.

By examining the lymph nodes for presence of cancer cells, one can get a good indication of whether the tumor has begun to spread from the colon to the rest of the body.

Microscopic view of colon wall

WHAT IS COLORECTAL CANCER?

All organs in the body are made of cells. Individual cells are so small, they can be seen only through a microscope. Normally, cells divide in an orderly fashion to replace cells that have aged and died. Controls within each cell tell it to stop dividing if no new cells are needed.

Occasionally, damage to DNA during cell duplication may cause the controls to malfunction. Cells begin to divide uncontrollably, forming lumps or tumors.

Tumors

The word "tumor" comes from a Latin word that means "swelling." A tumor is made up of cells that divide excessively, but do not invade other organs. For example, a fibroid in the uterus, or a fibroadenoma in the breast. These are called *benign*, that is, non-cancerous tumors.

Malignant tumors are composed of aggressively dividing cells that destroy surrounding tissues or travel to other parts of the body. Generally, the word "tumor" refers to a malignant condition, or cancer. Each cancer is named according to where it originated. So cancer that started in the colon, but has spread to the liver is still called colon cancer.

Polyps

Most cases of colon cancer arise from *polyps*—small growths on the lining of the colon. Colon polyps are benign (not cancerous) when they first appear, but some types of polyps can grow and become cancerous over time.

The polyps most likely to become cancerous are called **adenomas**. These polyps are made of glandular cells found in your colon lining. About 95% of all cases of colon cancer develop from adenomatous polyps.

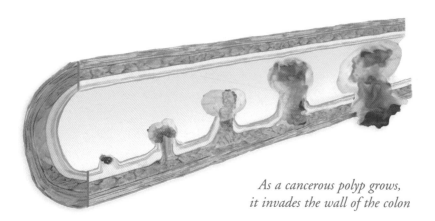

As a cancerous polyp grows, it invades the wall of the colon

It may take a polyp years to change from adenoma to cancer. The larger the polyp, the older it probably is, and the higher the risk that it contains a cancer. That is why it is so important to check the colon at regular intervals for presence of polyps, and to remove them as soon as possible.

Colorectal Cancer

If left untreated, polyps will often become cancerous. Cancer can also arise as a flat, non-polypoid lesion on the surface of the bowel. Cancer can grow in any part of the colon. This is called **colon cancer**. At least half of all cases occur in the left side of the large intestine.

When the cancer involves the rectum, it is called **rectal cancer**. Usually the two types are jointly called **colorectal** cancer.

HOW CANCER SPREADS

The earliest stage of colon cancer is called *carcinoma in situ*, which means "in place." If you have carcinoma in situ, the cancer is limited (localized) to the glands in the mucosa. Carcinoma in situ does not have the ability to spread to lymph nodes or to other areas of the body.

In the more advanced stages of colon cancer, called *invasive carcinoma*, the tumor penetrates into the colon wall. At this point, the cancer is positioned to spread to lymph nodes and to other organs in the pelvis and abdomen.

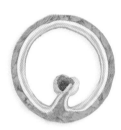

In situ cancer

Cancer cells that enter the lymph nodes can be carried to other parts of the body through the lymph system and form new tumors called **metastases**.

Most often, colon cancer spreads to the liver, but it can also spread to the ovaries, lungs, or brain. Colon cancer tends to spread to the liver first, because all of the blood from the colon drains to the liver before proceeding to the rest of the body. The management of metastatic cancer is more difficult and can involve many combinations of surgery and chemotherapy.

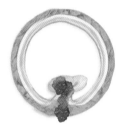

Invasive cancer

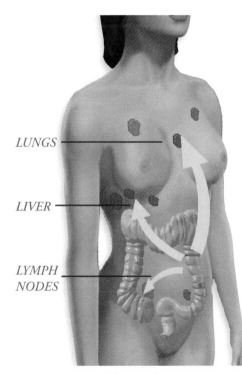

LUNGS

LIVER

LYMPH
NODES

Metastatic cancer

NOTES

CHAPTER 3

DIAGNOSIS AND STAGING

DIAGNOSIS

The only sure way to determine whether a tumor is malignant is to take a sample of the tumor and examine it under the microscope. This procedure is called a *biopsy*.

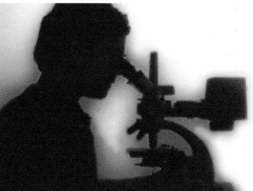

When abnormal growths are found during a sigmoidoscopy or colonoscopy, they can usually be biopsied immediately. This is done through the same instrument being used for the examination. The tissue samples obtained during the biopsy are sent to be examined under a microscope by a pathologist—a specialist in tumor identification.

Odds are that if you are reading this book, you already may have had a biopsy that showed your tumor was malignant. This would have been communicated to your physician through a *pathologist's report*.

PATHOLOGIST'S REPORT

A pathologist's report will usually include the following information:

Polyp site—where in the bowel it was found.

Polyp size—the larger, the greater the possibility of cancer.

Polyp configuration—the general shape of the poly. Polyps with a stalk are less suspicious than those without.

Histologic type—the type of cells in the tumor. Adenocarcinoma is the most common type of cell in colon cancer.

Histologic grade—how different the cancer cells look from normal cells is a good indication of how aggressive ("bad") they are.

Invasion—how deeply the cancer penetrates healthy tissue.

Assuming you go on to have surgery on the cancer, the surgeon will send whatever portion of colon or rectum is removed to the pathologist, who will then create a final report. This report will specify the size of the tumor, the type of cells, and the status of the tumor edges, or *margins*. Presence of cancerous cells near the edges is an indication that some cancer might have been left behind. The report will also specify whether cancer cells have reached the lymph nodes.

ADDITIONAL TESTS

At this point, you will probably have additional tests that will help your physician determine the type of treatment that will be most effective.

Why more tests? A biopsy can confirm that the diagnosis is cancer, but it will not show whether the cancer has spread to other parts of the body. This information is vital, because it will help determine what kind of treatment is called for to achieve the best results possible in your particular case.

The tests may include:

Chest x-rays
Tumors that have spread to the lungs can often be seen on chest x-rays.

Blood tests
Carcinoembryonic antigen (CEA) is a protein that is produced by colon cancer cells. Currently, doctors measure a person's CEA level before and after surgery to help determine whether the procedure has completely removed the cancer. After surgery, your CEA level should be normal. If your CEA level increases steadily after surgery, it may be an indication that the cancer has returned.

Liver function tests will assess the function of the liver—a common site for colon cancer spread.

PET Scan

PET scans use small amounts of radioactive tracer and a special camera to obtain information about tissue function. The resulting images help physicians distinguish metastases from normal tissue, and play a very important part in tumor staging.

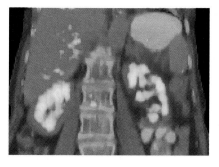

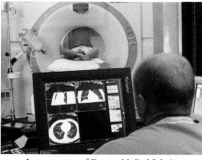

Image courtesy of Siemens Medical Solutions

CT Scan

CAT scan, CT scan, or Computerized Axial Tomography all mean the same thing. This test uses ordinary x-rays, and a rotating film/source system to obtain detailed, three dimensional images of your body. The test is painless and takes less than an hour.

MRI Scan

MRI or Magnetic Resonance Imaging uses a combination of magnetic energy and ordinary radio waves to create images of the inside of your body. It is generally not done unless the CT scan was indefinite, or there is a need to see the liver better.

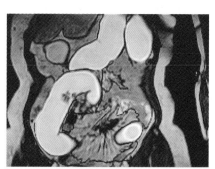

Image courtesy of Siemens Medical Solutions

Because the MRI unit can feel cramped, notify the technologist or your physician if you feel uncomfortable in confined spaces. MRI is painless, and does not expose you to x-ray radiation. The test takes about an hour.

STAGING

The process of analyzing all the pertinent information and assigning your disease to a particular group, or stage, is called *staging*.

Not all colorectal cancers will be treated the same way. The therapy will be adjusted to each individual cancer and situation. To help determine who should get what treatment, cancer specialists rely on staging—a system that places the cancer into a certain group. The stage of your tumor is the most important factor in deciding what type of treatment is best for you.

Clinical staging is the initial and tentative staging that is based on the results of the physical exam and the diagnostic tests performed before surgery. These may include others such as liver function tests to make sure the liver is functioning well and a chest x-ray to make sure the tumor has not spread to the lungs.

The final determination of the stage, called *pathological staging*, will come after the surgeon had an opportunity to examine the inside of the abdomen during the procedure, and the tumor has been removed surgically and examined under a microscope.

TNM

Today, the TNM—tumor, node, metastasis—staging system, which places patients into one of four stages (Stage I-IV), is the common method. This system is based on: the depth of invasion of the tumor; the presence of cancer cells in the lymph nodes; and metastasis, or spread, to other organs.

Tumor depth of invasion (T) is determined when the tumor is removed and sent to the pathologist.

Lymph nodes (N) are checked for tumor spread at the time of surgery. A minimum of twelve nodes is needed for an accurate assessment.

Metastasis, or spread to other organs (M), is assessed with x-rays, scans, and blood tests.

QUESTIONS TO ASK
YOUR DOCTOR:

- **What stage is my cancer?**

- **How far has my cancer spread?**

- **What other tests do I need?**

- **Will the stage be changed after the surgery?**

- **How often do you get at least twelve lymph nodes for examination during surgery?**

The pathologist will examine the specimen removed during surgery, review other information, and assign a rating to each of the three letters.

The exact rating is very detailed. For example T1 is a cancer that has grown through the muscularis mucosa and extends into the submucosa. A T4b cancer has grown through the wall of the colon or rectum and is attached to or invades nearby tissues. N1b means cancer cells are found in two to three nearby lymph nodes. And M1a indicates that the cancer has spread to 1 distant organ or set of distant lymph nodes.

All the ratings are assembled to determine the stage of the tumor. For example, a T1 tumor (one that has not spread beyond the submucosa layer of the bowel), that is N0 (no nodes have been invaded by cancer) and M0 (there is no evidence of spread to other organs) is labeled T1 N0 M0. By refering to staging tables, this tumor is staged as stage I.

The stage, in turn will guide the medical team in selecting the appropriate therapy. The extent of the treatment will be matched to the extent of spread of the disease. The more extensive the spread, the more intense the treatment.

You may find it helpful to think of stage as degree of risk presented by a particular tumor. At one end of the scale are the low-risk situations: very tiny tumors that have not spread through the bowel wall. Further along are slightly larger tumors that have penetrated the bowel wall. At the other end of the scale are tumors that have invaded the lymph nodes or spread to other parts of the body.

If you are at the low risk end of the scale, your treatment may require only surgical removal of the tumor. More advanced tumors may be treated with more extensive surgery and aggressive additional therapy. The next chapter goes into greater detail about making treatment choices.

Stage Groupings According to TNM Staging *

Stage 0: Tis, N0, M0
The cancer is in the earliest stage, carcinoma in situ.

Stage I: T1 N0 M0; T2 N0 M0
Cancer has begun to spread, but has not spread to nearby lymph nodes.

Stage IIA: T3 N0 M0
The cancer has grown into the outermost layers of the bowel.

Stage IIB: T4a N0 M0
The cancer has grown through the wall of the colon or rectum.

Stage IIC: T4b N0 M0
Cancer has spread to other organs near the colon or rectum. It has not reached the lymph nodes.

Stage IIIA: T1-T2, N1, M0
Spread to the lymph nodes, but not to distant parts of the body.

Stage IIIB: T3-T4a, N1, M0 or T2-T3, N2a, M0 or T1-T2, N2b, M0
Cancer has grown into the outermost layers but has not reached nearby organs.

Stage IIIC: T4a, N2a, M0, or T3-T4a, N2b, M0, or T4b, N1-N2, M0
Cancer has reached nearby organs but has not spread to distant sites.

Stage IVA: any T, any N, M1a
Spread to one distant organ or one set of lymph nodes.

Stage IVB: any T, any N, M1b
Most advanced cancer that has spread to several distant parts of the body, such as liver and lungs.

This is a very simplified version. For a complete description, check out the latest American Joint Committee on Cancer (AJCC) staging information online.

CHAPTER 4

TREATMENT OPTIONS OVERVIEW

In this chapter we will offer you a bird's eye view of the various treatments available for colorectal cancer. In some cases of colorectal cancer, the treatment decision is very simple. No one would consider major surgery for a tiny polyp. Other decisions are much more complex, and present no clearly right or wrong choice. Choosing the most appropriate cancer treatment is a decision that ideally involves the patient, the family, and the healthcare team. By getting acquainted with the issues, you will be able to participate more actively in the decision process.

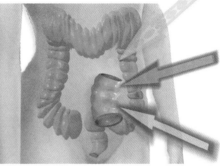

TREATMENT TYPES

The goal of colorectal cancer treatment is to eliminate all the cancer cells present in the body: that is, to cure the cancer. This includes the obvious cells within the tumor itself, and the undetectable cells (micrometastases) that may have broken off the main tumor and traveled to other parts of the body, where they will be a threat later on.

Treatment that targets cancer in the location where it was first found—the *primary site*—is called *local therapy*. Treatment that can reach all parts of the body to eliminate runaway cells is called *systemic treatment*. Because this type of treatment is often given as an addition, or an adjunct to the main local therapy, it is also called *adjuvant therapy*. When additional therapy is given before the main therapy, (for example, radiation therapy to pre-shrink a tumor before surgery) it is referred to as *neo-adjuvant therapy*.

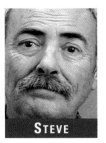

STEVE

When I first heard the different words—colectomy, colostomy, chemo… I was so confused, I didn't know where to start. Eventually I got the hang of it, so I could keep up with the explanations.

Sometimes the goal of treatment is not to cure the disease, but to decrease the effects of the disease on the body—for example, to achieve pain relief. In this case the treatment is called *palliative therapy.*

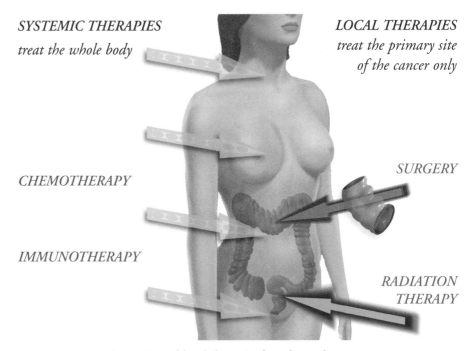

Systemic and local therapies for colorectal cancer

SURGERY

Surgery is the main form of therapy for most types of colorectal cancer. The goal is to remove the tumor and cure the cancer. Surgery generally removes the entire tumor with an area of healthy tissue around it to ensure no cancerous cells are left behind.

If the cancer is in the colon, the procedure will involve the removal of the tumor and adjacent lymph nodes. This is called *colorectal resection.* If the cancer is in the rectum, surgery may involve *local* or *transanal excision* of the tumor.

A new surgical approach is now available: *minimally invasive surgery*, or MIS. It is described in detail in Chapter 7.

Colorectal Resection

If the cancer is larger, if it is located above the rectum, or it has spread beyond the first layer of the bowel, a local excision may not be an option, because it will probably leave tumor cells behind. A more complex operation is required. This will entail the removal of a segment of the colon, with the cancer and a small length of healthy bowel around it. A procedure called an *anastomosis* will usually be done to reconnect the parts of the large intestine to each other.

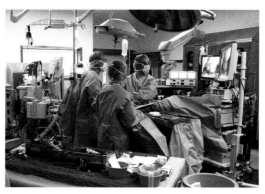

Minimally invasive colon surgery

If the cancer is located in the rectum, you may be treated with radiation therapy to shrink the tumor and make the operation less challenging.

On the rare occasion when the two ends of the colon cannot be sewn back together, a stoma (opening) is made connecting the bowel to the outside of the body, so that waste can pass through into a bag. This is called a *colostomy*. It may or may not be permanent, depending on the case. You may want to read the "Colostomy" section in Chapter 8, and seek a second opinion before agreeing to have a colostomy done.

Transanal Resection

If the cancer is in the rectum, if it is found to be early stage (T1 or T2), and if it has not spread, the surgeon may be able to remove it using a *transanal resection*. This procedure is done through the anus, without cutting through the wall of the abdomen. See Chapter 8 for details.

CHEMOTHERAPY

Chemotherapy uses drugs that can reach all parts of the body to stop the growth of cancer cells, either by killing them or by stopping the cells from dividing. Chemotherapy is taken by mouth or injected into a vein or muscle. Sometimes chemotherapy drugs are placed directly into the abdomen, where they can have a more direct effect on escaped cancer cells. Chemotherapy is an *adjuvant systemic* treatment.

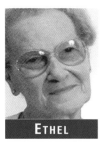

ETHEL

I liked looking at all the options. I actually made up little charts, little doodles, to help me keep things organized in my head. It's nice to know why they are recommending what they are... Call me a control freak, but hey, it is my body...

RADIATION THERAPY

Radiation therapy uses high-energy x-rays to kill cancer cells. There are two types of radiation therapy. External beam radiation therapy, or EBRT, uses a machine to send a radiation beam through the area from where the cancer was removed. EBRT is sometimes used before surgery to shrink the tumor. Brachytherapy uses a radioactive substance sealed in needles, seeds, wires, or catheters that are placed directly into or near the cancer site.

Both are considered *local adjuvant therapies* and are designed to ensure that no cancer cells remain behind at the site of the tumor. Radiation therapy is covered in Chapter 10.

TREATMENT SELECTION

Which treatment, or combination of treatments, is right for you? The answer depends on many factors, including:

• The stage of your cancer (whether the cancer has spread, and if so, what other parts of your body are affected.)

• Your age and general health (health problems in addition to colon cancer may make certain treatments more risky for you.)

• Your feelings about the treatments available to you and their possible long- and short-term side effects.

Remember that generally there is no rush to come to a conclusion. Take the time—a few weeks if you need to—to learn whatever you want to know about the treatment. Discuss your concerns with the healthcare team. Consider using a friend or a loved one as a sounding board. Interview other patients who have undergone the treatment you are contemplating. Then make your decision.

CHAPTER 5

SURGERY –
POLYPECTOMY OR LOCAL EXCISION

To ensure the best chance for successful treatment, it is important to remove the entire tumor, using the most direct approach possible. That means some type of surgery. Other treatments, such as radiation therapy or chemotherapy, cannot replace surgery, although in some cases they may play an important role in the treatment process.

There are two types of surgical procedures for removing cancerous tumors from the colon or rectum.

If the tumor is small and hasn't invaded the layers of the colon, it is possible to remove just the tumor, with a safety margin of healthy tissue around it, without cutting all the way through (transecting) the bowel. This is called *local excision*, *polypectomy*, or *transanal excision*, and is used primarily for very early polyps and for early cancers in the rectum.

If the tumor has begun to infiltrate—or spread—across the wall, then the best option is to remove the tumor in a procedure called a *partial* or *segmental colectomy*. In this case, the section of the colon containing the tumor is removed, together with a short piece of healthy bowel on either side, and the ends reconnected.

In this chapter we will discuss *polypectomy* or *local excision*.

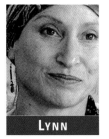

LYNN

The good news—if there was any good news—is that the doctor was able to take out the whole thing right during colonoscopy, so when he got the report back and it said "malignant" the thing was already out.

QUESTIONS TO ASK YOUR
ANESTHESIOLOGIST:

• Will you give me some-
thing to help me relax
before the procedure?

• How long will it take
me to get back to nor-
mal after the sedation?

• What are the side effects
of sedation?

LOCAL EXCISION

Tumors that have not spread beyond the inner layers of the bowel lining (mucosa), can sometimes be treated without major surgery. There are two ways to perform the local excision:

In case of colon tumors (polyps), the physician can remove them with a sigmoidoscope or colonoscope (the same devices that are used to view the colon lining during a diagnostic examination) without cutting through the colon or through the abdominal wall. This procedure is called a *local excision* or *polypectomy*.

For rectal polyps, or some very early rectal cancers, a colorectal surgeon can remove the tumor and a margin of healthy tissue by operating through the anus. This is called a *transanal resection*.

Because it is so important to eliminate all of the cancerous tissue, local resection is not an option for treating cancers that cannot be completely removed with this procedure. Your physician will consider the cancer's size and its exact location, and review the biopsy results to decide whether a local resection is the right choice for you.

Before Surgery

To ensure the speedy completion of the procedure, it is important that your bowel is as clean as possible. If you had a colonoscopy before, you are already familiar with the bowel preparation, or "prep."

Specific prep instructions vary from physician to physician. More than likely, you'll need to be on a clear liquid diet for a short time. That means no solid foods, and not even milk. Broth and Jell-O are acceptable.

The night before the procedure you will take a potent laxative, followed by a large amount of fluids. You will probably finish off with an enema on the morning of your surgery. In some cases, this step is not done.

It is imperative that you follow the instructions given to you. A poorly cleaned colon may require the procedure to be postponed, or can result in polyps or small tumors being missed.

You'll also be asked to sign an informed consent form as an indication that you understand the procedure and the possible complications, such as infection and bleeding. Read the form carefully and ask for explanations of any parts that you are not comfortable with.

A local excision can be done in an outpatient surgicenter or in a hospital. When you arrive at the facility, you may be given additional enemas to complete the cleaning of your colon. You will be asked to remove dentures or glasses. If you wear contact lenses, make arrangements for their safekeeping. Do not wear makeup or jewelry on the day of your procedure.

The Procedure

A polypectomy may be done by a gastroenterologist (a doctor who specializes in diagnosing and treating diseases of the digestive tract) or by a colorectal surgeon.

The actual removal of the lesion itself is painless because the bowel nerves are only sensitive to stretching. You will be given medication to make you drowsy and comfortable, and you probably won't even remember much about the procedure.

You will be positioned comfortably on your side, with your knees slightly bent. The physician will insert the colonoscope into your anus, and using a TV monitor will gradually advance the instrument up the colon, carefully examining the wall as the tube travels upward.

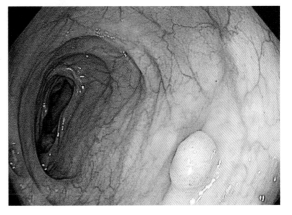

Polyp as seen through a colonoscope

When the tip of the colonoscope reaches the suspect area, the physician will identify and remove the polyp.

If the lesion is shaped like a mushroom, the excision is done by passing a wire snare down the colonoscope, looping it around the stalk, and tightening the snare. Then an electric current is passed through the wire. This coagulates the blood vessels and cuts through the stalk.

QUESTIONS TO ASK
YOUR DOCTOR:

• How much pain should I expect after the procedure?

• How long before I can go back to my regular work or leisure activities?

• What follow up visits do you recommend?

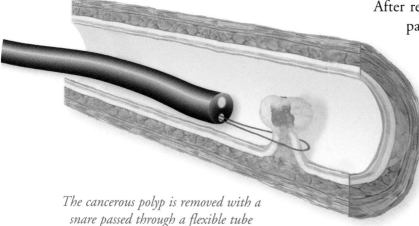

The cancerous polyp is removed with a snare passed through a flexible tube

After removal, the polyp is sent to the pathology laboratory for microscopic examination. If the cancer is a superficial lesion (shaped like a mound, rather than the usual mushroom), the physician will use other tools to remove the cancerous tissue from the surface of the bowel, being careful not to leave cancerous cells behind.

Transanal Excision

For select, very early rectal cancers, your surgeon may recommend a *transanal excision.* Transanal excision involves cutting through layers of the rectum to remove the cancer, as well as some surrounding normal rectal tissue. The procedure can be done through the anus, and leaves the rectum itself intact.

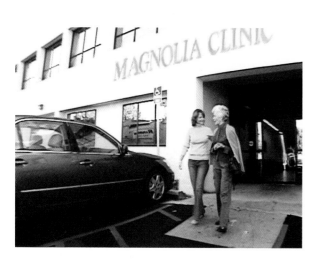

Ask a friend or relative to drive you home

After the Procedure

Following a *polypectomy,* you will remain in the recovery area for about an hour. The length of time you will be at the clinic varies for each patient. It depends on the bowel preparation, the procedure and your recovery time. The average procedure and recovery time is about two hours.

Your doctor will discuss the results of your examination before you leave the recovery room. You may want a family member present when the doctor discusses these results, since your memory might still be affected by the medication you received prior to the procedure.

You will be given specific instructions to follow, and a list of symptoms for which you should call the physician.

Because it may take a while for you to be fully awake enough to drive a car, you will need a friend or relative to accompany you to the hospital to drive you home after the procedure.

If you have a *transanal excision*, your recovery and discharge may be different from what you could have expected if you had a polypectomy.

A transanal excision is often performed in a hospital, under general anesthesia. Depending on the extent of the excision and your health, you may need to stay one or more nights in the hospital.

If your tumor is removed by either polypectomy or transanal excision, it is very important to remember that depending upon what the pathology repost says, your physicians may recommend further treatment, such as radiation therapy, chemotherapy, or more extensive surgery.

Side Effects

As with any surgical procedure, there are risks associated with local excision and polypectomy.

Before surgery, your physician will describe to you in detail the complications that are possible given your particular health situation.

One possible but rare complication of local resection is perforation of the bowel. This may require surgery, probably through the wall of the abdomen.

Sometimes there is prolonged bleeding from the excision site, but the bleeding generally stops with no additional surgery. In any case, don't hesitate to call your physician if you experience any symptoms that you didn't expect.

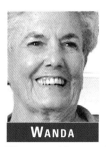

WANDA

The worst thing was the darn'd enemas—at home, then at the surgicenter. The rest was a piece of cake. My husband drove me home. It is really nothing as operations go. Other than, of course, you have cancer… But I'm thankful I didn't have the surgical scar to deal with.

NOTES

CHAPTER 6

SURGERY –
OPEN COLON RESECTION

The local excision or polypectomy discussed in the preceding chapter is a good option for very early cancers that have not invaded the wall of the colon. But if the tumor is large, or has invaded the bowel wall, you will need a more extensive surgical procedure.

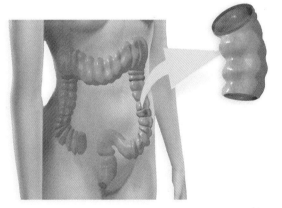

Colon resection, *colectomy*, or *partial colectomy* are different names given to a type of surgery that consist of removing a part, or all, of the colon. This is the most common approach to treating large polyps or cancers that have grown into the wall of the colon.

Unlike a polypectomy which can be performed in an outpatient facility by a gastroenterologist, colon resection is done in a hospital operating room, by a surgeon.

If the tumor is in the rectum and is full thickness (T3 or T4) or has spread to lymph nodes, your physician may recommend *neoadjuvant treatment*—radiation therapy along with chemotherapy before surgery—in order to shrink the tumor so it can be removed more effectively, and decrease the chance of a permanent colostomy.

An exciting development is the introduction of *laparoscopic surgery* and *robotic-assisted surgery*. Both of these techniques offer several important advantages over conventional, or open, colectomy. They are described in a later chapter.

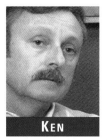

KEN

Sure, you can get used to it. But still, it cramps your style. So the happiest day, other than finding out the cancer was totally removed, was the day they closed my colostomy.

FACING SURGERY

Understandably, the prospect of facing major surgery might be daunting. To ease your anxiety, you may want to talk to other patients who had the same type of surgery, and learn from their experiences.

Before Surgery Checklist

Stop smoking and using recreational drugs as soon as possible.

Stop drinking alcohol.

Stop all medications that interfere with blood clotting, such as aspirin containing medications, a week before surgery. This includes Advil, Motrin, etc..

Discuss with your internist the stoppage of blood thinners like Coumadin.

Stop taking vitamins, unless you clear them with the surgeon or the surgical nurse.

Check your health and disability benefits and schedule time off.

Recruit help—even simple household chores may be more than you can handle for a while after surgery.

Consider banking your own blood for possible transfusions.

Make sure you discussed with your surgeon whether you are a candidate for the Minimally Invasive Surgery option. (See Chapter 7)

Most importantly, try to concentrate on the thought that surgery is the best way to cure colorectal cancer. In other words, you are taking the step that will give you the best chance of successful treatment. Before long the discomfort of surgery will be gone and the incisions will be healed, and you will have the satisfaction of knowing that you took the best step toward a total cure.

For a colectomy, just as for the polypectomy or transanal excision described earlier, your colon needs to be as clean as possible. The need for such cleansing has been recently debated, but there are advantages to you and the surgeon.

Your surgeon will give you specific prep instructions. More than likely, they will include being on a clear liquid diet for two days, and a potent laxative, followed by a large amount of fluids the night before the procedure. In addition, you may be started on some antibiotics to remove as much bacteria from your colon as possible.

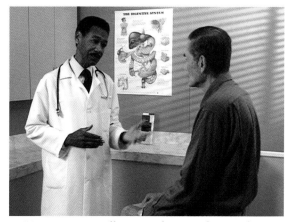

Your surgeon will review the procedure with you before your scheduled surgery

Sometimes colon surgery requires a blood transfusion, especially if you are already anemic prior to the operation. If you want to avoid receiving blood bank products, ask your surgeon about donating and storing your own blood before surgery.

On the day of the surgery, you'll first go through an admission process at the hospital. Your surgeon will have already reviewed with you all aspects of the procedure, and the possible risks and complications. The hospital staff will ask you to sign an informed consent form.

Informed Consent Form

- You understand the type of the procedure and the purpose for it.
- The risks of the surgery and the anesthetic have been explained to you.
- You understand that intravenous medication, including drugs, anesthesia, and blood transfusions, will be administered.
- Any tissue removed during surgery may be examined and disposed.

- If I have general anesthesia, how long will it take me to get back to normal?

- Will you give me something to control the pain after I wake up from the anesthetic?

Make sure you feel comfortable with what you are signing. If there is anything that you don't understand, ask to see your doctor.

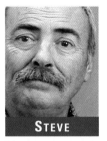

STEVE

I had my surgery through tubes. The doctors don't cut the skin, just make holes. From what I hear, I had it much easier after surgery. I was back out tinkering in the yard... Probably in a less than a week or so...

After you check in, an anesthesiologist or a nurse anesthetist will meet with you and select a general anesthetic that is best suited to your medical condition. Before they can make a recommendation, they need to know about all aspects of your health. The anesthesia team will ask you about:

- Your medical history and any problems with your heart or lungs.
- Current conditions such as skin infections, colds, or tooth decay.
- Allergies to medications or food.
- Prescriptions, over-the-counter medications, or drugs that you may be taking, including herbal supplements.
- Smoking and drinking patterns.

Once you are in the staging area, the anesthesiologist will start an intravenous line (an "IV") in one of your arms, and perhaps give you something to help you relax.

The Surgical Procedure

When the surgical team is ready, you will be taken to the operating room. Several devices will be attached to you, such as an automatic blood pressure cuff, a heart monitor, and a blood oxygen monitor.

The anesthesiologist will inject a drug into your vein through the tubing, and you will fall asleep almost immediately. A tube will be placed in your throat to maintain a clear way for you to breathe during the surgery. Your blood pressure, pulse, and breathing will be closely monitored during the entire procedure. Afterwords, you will be placed on antibiotics.

THINGS TO TAKE WITH YOU TO THE HOSPITAL

Nightgown or pajamas

Slippers

Toiletries

Shaving utensils

Books or iPod

Favorite pillow

Warm socks

Change of clothing for going home

An open partial colectomy takes between one and four hours. The operation involves making an incision through your abdominal wall and removing the part of your colon containing the cancer, along with a short section of normal colon tissue surrounding the tumor.

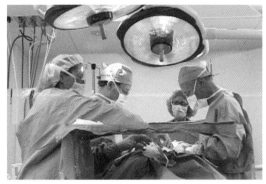

A surgical team in the operating room

In addition, the surgeon will remove all of the lymph nodes near the part of the colon affected by the cancer. Both the segment of colon and the lymph nodes will be sent to the pathologist for examination under a microscope for evidence of tumor spread.

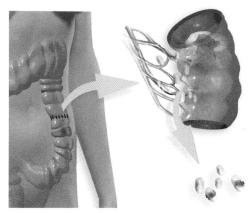

In particular, the pathologist will verify that no cancer cells are found near the cut margins of the specimen—ideally no closer than half an inch. If cancer cells extend to the margin, there may be a possibility that some of the tumor was left behind, and you may need additional treatment.

The lymph nodes near the tumor will be examined for evidence of tumor spread

If cancer cells are found within the lymph nodes, then it is possible that the tumor has begun to spread to other organs. In this case, your healthcare team will discuss the possibility of adding a systemic treatment, such as chemotherapy, to the surgical treatment.

In most cases, the surgeon will reconnect the remaining ends of your colon together (this is called anastomosis) so stool can pass out of your body in the usual way.

Risks and Complications

As with any surgical procedure, there are risks associated with colon resection. In general, these include the following: Your surgeon will describe to you in detail the procedure and the complications that are possible.

- Reaction to anesthesia
- Blood clots
- Bleeding from the operative site into the abdomen
- Infections, including pneumonia and formation of an abscess inside the abdomen or the colon
- Bowel content leakage into the abdomen
- Injury to other structures in the abdomen
- Formation of a fistula—an unwanted connection between the skin and the intestines.

- **How much colon will be removed?**

- **How will the colectomy affect my eating?**

- **Where, and how big, will the scar be?**

- **Do I qualify for Minimally Invasive Surgery?**

- **How much pain should I expect in the first few days after the procedure?**

- **How long before I can go back to my regular work or leisure activities?**

- **Will there be any long term effects?**

- **Will you be sending tissues for molecular testing?**

Will I Need a Colostomy?

A colostomy is a procedure that creates a connection between the bowel and the outside of the abdomen, so stool can pass through and be collected into a bag attached to the skin of the abdomen.

The issue of a colostomy is a major concern for most patients. In general, a colostomy is required only if the cancer is in the lower rectum and the anus needs to be removed.

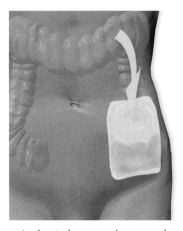

If you required an urgent operation, a temporary colostomy may also be necessary due to your condition or the condition of your large intestine at that time.

With today's advances in early diagnosis and improved treatment of colorectal cancer, most patients being treated for cancer that is in the colon, rather than the rectum, will not need a permanent or temporary colostomy.

A plastic bag attaches over the colostomy site to collect feces

RECOVERY AFTER OPEN COLECTOMY

After surgery, you'll be taken to the recovery room. As you wake up from the anesthetic, you may feel cold, and your throat may be sore from the tube used for anesthesia. You may fade between waking and sleeping for several hours.

You will have a tube in your urethra, called a Folley catheter, to help you urinate after surgery. This tube will be removed within a few days. You will not need a tube in your nose, called an NG tube.

Most patients like to have a friend or relative meet them after the operation. You can ask your surgeon how long it will take before you will be brought to your room after surgery, and to arrange with the hospital to allow that person to meet you there.

To avoid overstressing your bowels, for the first 24-48 hours you will be restricted to sips of water. Your surgeon will be looking for your ability to pass gas from your rectum as an indication that your bowels are recovering and starting to move normally. Generally, you will soon be allowed to eat more substantial fare such as soups and applesauce.

Each patient reacts to surgery differently. Most patients will stay in the hospital for four to seven days after an open colectomy.

What determines how long you will stay in the hospital? Your medical team will want to be sure of three things: that you can tolerate a normal diet, that you can ambulate independently, and that your pain can be controlled with oral medications. Get a passing grade on all three, and you will be free to go home.

One of the usual side effects of surgery and anesthesia is partial blockage or collapse of the breathing sacs within the lungs. Someone on your healthcare team will teach you how to do breathing exercises. Their purpose is to force your lungs to re-expand. Be diligent about these breathing exercises—they will help speed your recovery. Continue them even after you go home.

You will probably have incision pain for days after surgery. Do not hesitate to take the pain medications prescribed. Accepting pain unnecessarily leads to added fatigue, prevents you from breathing freely, and may interfere with healing. This is a case where the saying "No pain, no gain" does not apply.

One of the most common concerns to most patients undergoing surgery is fatigue—a feeling of tiredness. You too will probably feel more tired than usual for a while. Don't be discouraged. You've just been through general anesthesia and major surgery, and less than perfect performance is to be expected. Do not push yourself. When your body has recovered, your energy will return on its own.

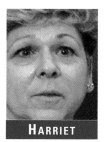

HARRIET

That surgery, it took the wind out of my sails. My husband had to do everything for me for two weeks, maybe longer. Every time I'd get up, I felt like lying back down again. It was a good month before I was back to my normal self.

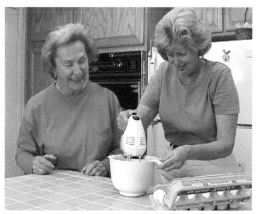

Enlist the help of your friends

As soon as you can, start a walking program. Walking is probably one of the best exercises for you at this time. It helps to keep blood clots from forming in your legs, improves bowel function, and returns your lungs to their pre-surgery state.

It is normal to expect to be limited to taking sponge baths for a few days after surgery so that your incision can heal. Most patients will be ready for a shower prior to leaving the hospital. Follow your surgeon's instructions on changing bandages. When showering, gently wash around the incision, and don't take a bath until your wound closes completely.

Immediately after surgery, you'll probably have trouble moving. Use your body as tolerated, but avoid active movements until you get your doctor's approval. Don't be afraid to enlist the help of a friend or relative until your strength returns.

Many people return to normal activities within four to six weeks. If your job requires heavy lifting or strenuous physical work, you may need to change your activities until you have fully regained your strength.

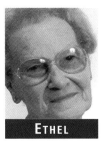

ETHEL

When I left the hospital I had a colostomy, but the cancer was gone. I felt like a brand new person, with a new lease on life. When you have a brush with death, what is a little inconvenience like a colostomy for a few weeks.

Before you decide to have surgery to treat colon cancer, make sure you understand the following:

- What kind of surgery will be done.
- What you need to do to prepare for the surgery.
- How long it will take for you to recover from the surgery.
- The possible risks and complications associated with the surgery.
- What additional treatment you may need after surgery.
- How the surgery may affect your daily activities.
- The cost of the surgery and the drugs, treatments, and hospital stay associated with the surgery.
- Who will pay for the surgery and its associated costs.

DIET

You may have a consultation with a dietitian before you go home from the hospital. You will be told to drink at least eight glasses of water a day to stay hydrated.

Most patients who have had colon surgery find that their bowel habits have changed. This may include softer or more frequent stools. These changes can generally be managed with medications or with bulking agents and improve with time.

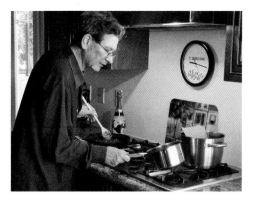

A bowel management program may be as simple as slowing down your digestion process by avoiding large meals or hot liquids at meal time, or by retraining the colon to empty itself fully at a specific time during the day that is convenient for you. Your healthcare team will give you specific instructions to help make sure that colon surgery has a minimal impact on your quality of life.

The right diet will help relieve many of the side effects of colon surgery

Metastatic Cancer – Liver Surgery

Sometimes during the initial evaluation of a case, or during surgery on the colon, the surgeon will find that the cancer has spread (metastasized).

Both colon and rectal cancers spread to the lungs, but they are more likely to spread to the liver.

If the metastases are small and few, the surgeon may recommend an operation to remove the affected part of the liver with the goal of curing the disease, or extending life expectancy. This surgical approach to metastatic cancer is always combined with chemotherapy treatment, which is described in a later chapter.

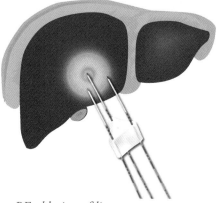

RF ablation of liver metastases

The preferred procedure is to perform a ***partial liver resection***—in other words, to remove part of the liver. If this is not possible because of the number or location of the metastases, or for reasons of your general health, then an alternative approach is cryosurgery or radiofrequency ablation.

Cryosurgery destroys the cancer tissues by freezing them with supercooled thin probes inserted directly into the metastases.

Radiofrequency ablation (also referred to as RFA) destroys the cancer tissue by heating it with small probes inserted into the metastases.

Recovery after liver surgery is sometimes more difficult than after a colectomy. Your healthcare team to review the details with you.

MINIMALLY INVASIVE SURGERY

Surgery offers the best opportunities for curing colorectal cancer. But long incisions and extensive manipulation of the bowel during surgical procedures do take a toll in terms of post-operative pain and recovery time.

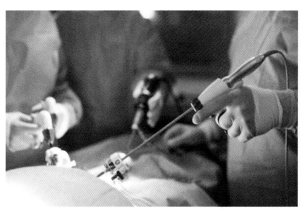

To reduce these adverse effects, surgeons and manufacturers of surgical instruments have teamed up to develop techniques that can reach and remove a tumor with as little intrusion into the abdominal cavity as possible.

Today the techniques include *laporoscopic surgery*, and *robotic-assisted surgery*. Both are performed through small incisions, and therefore are called *minimally invasive*.

Image courtesy of Ethicon Endo-Surgery

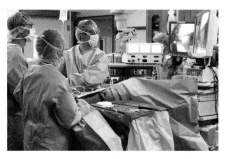

Surgeons operate by watching their work on monitors

You may want to review the chapters that describe the more conventional (open) procedures, in order to get a better point of comparison, and to review the suggested questions. Many of the questions to ask apply to all surgical chapters.

LAPAROSCOPIC SURGERY

Instead of long incisions and a surgeon's hands to perform conventional surgery, *laparoscopic surgery* relies on a few very small incisions, and several delicate instruments, thus creating a smaller impact on the body. For this reason, laparoscopic surgery is also referred to as *minimally invasive surgery*, or *MIS*.

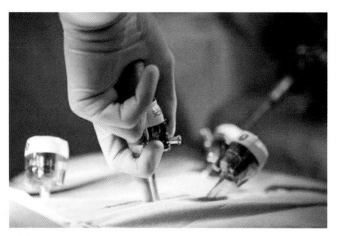

Trocars, or ports, are used to insert endoscopic instruments
Image courtesy of Ethicon Endo-Surgery

The preparation and anesthesia for laparoscopic surgery is the same as was described earlier in the open surgery chapter. When you are properly anesthetized, the surgeon will make several small incisions in the skin. The incisions will be 5-12mm (about a quarter to half an inch). Some of these incisions will be used to inject carbon dioxide into the abdomen. This will push the abdominal wall away from the intestine and allow the surgeon to work.

Special tubes, called trocars, or ports, will be used to insert delicate tools, including a viewing device called a laparoscope, and to perform the surgery.

The surgical team will operate by manipulating the instruments from outside while watching their work on a high definition video monitor.

A laparoscopic colectomy is technically more challenging than open surgery. The procedure can take from two to four hours.

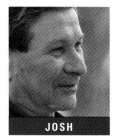

JOSH

First I took it easy. I have two grandchildren who I promised to babysit. So grandpa was able to run around with them. And when I went back to work three weeks later, they couldn't believe I already had the surgery.

Laparoscopic surgery of the rectum is even more difficult than laparoscopic colon surgery. The rectum sits in the narrow pelvis surrounded by tight bony structures and many important organs such as the bladder, the prostate or vagina, and the pelvic nerves that are responsible for proper sexual and urinary function. Because of this, laparoscopic surgery of the rectum can take three to six hours.

Benefits of Minimally Invasive Surgery

Many studies have shown that laparoscopic surgery offers many benefits when compared with traditional open surgery.

> ### Benefits of Minimally Invasive Surgery
>
> - Small incisions with reduced pain
> - Less blood loss and lower rate of transfusions
> - Reduced need of narcotic pain medication
> - A faster return of normal bowel function
> - Faster recovery, with fewer hospital days
> - Markedly higher quality of life

In some studies, the difference was impressive. For example, patients who underwent laparoscopic colectomy returned to their usual activity, on average, two weeks after surgery, whereas patients who underwent open colectomy reported returning to their usual activity seven weeks after surgery.

Overall, shorter recovery time with reduced narcotic use and quicker time to first bowel movement, oral intake, and normal diet translate into shorter hospital stays.

Risks and Complications

The rate of complications of laparoscopic colectomy is overall the same as for open surgery. The rates of wound infections and subsequent scar formation and hernia formation are all lower with a minimally invasive approach. The specific complications, such as bleeding, perforation, infections and others, have been discussed in an earlier chapter.

What is different about laparoscopic procedures is that they are quite demanding technically. The surgeon's experience is important, and there is a signif-

QUESTIONS TO ASK YOUR SURGEON:

- How many Minimally Invasive Surgery procedures of this type have you performed?
- What benefits can I expect in my particular case?
- Where, and how big, will the scars be?
- How much pain should I expect in the first few days after the procedure?
- How long before I can go back to my regular work or leisure activities?

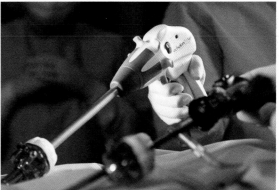

Endoscopic instruments offer convenient access to organs deep in the pelvis
Image courtesy of Ethicon Endo-Surgery

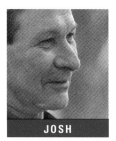

JOSH

The first thing I realized
when I came to was that I
didn't hurt. And now, two
weeks later, I don't feel like
I had surgery.

I thought, No way am I
going to get to go home in
three days – but come discharge day and, amazing, I
was fine to go.

icant learning curve. In the hands of a surgeon who has not received ade-
quate training, or hasn't yet performed a large number of these procedures, the complication rate may be significantly higher.

Since rectal surgery may be even more challenging than colon surgery, it
goes without saying that technical errors during rectal surgery can have
dramatic consequences on postoperative recovery and on your future.

If you are considering a laparoscopic procedure, you should find a surgeon
who has considerable experience with laparoscopic colon surgery before
agreeing to have the operation. It is helpful to assess a surgeon's expertise
by asking how many similar operations he or she typically performs in one
year, and whether he or she has published or given lectures in the field.

Although studies have shown that minimally invasive rectal surgery is safe
and results in better recovery compared with open rectal surgery, it must
be stressed that there are only a handful of centers around the country that
have sufficient experience with this approach.

Is Minimally Invasive Surgery Right for Me?

Unless there are specific reasons why a laparoscopic approach cannot be
performed, (these are rare: multiple prior operations for intra-abdominal
infection, tumors invading other organs) most
patients can be treated with laparoscopic surgery.
In the hands of the right surgeon, any segment of
the colon can be removed via a laparoscopy. Studies
have shown that even obese patients and patients
who have had prior surgery can have, and greatly
benefit from, minimally invasive surgery.

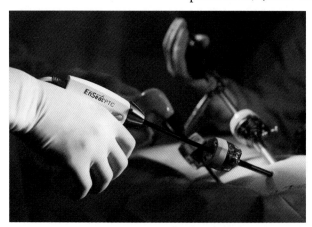

*Endoscopic instruments enable the surgical team
to operate from outside the body*

Image courtesy of Ethicon Endo-Surgery

Minimally invasive colorectal surgery is rapidly
becoming the standard of care for surgical treatment.
In 2005, 15% to 20% of colectomy procedures used
a minimally invasive approach. By 2014 it is project-
ed that 65% of colectomies will be performed laparo-
scopically.

ROBOTIC SURGERY

Robotic technology is the latest advance in minimally invasive surgery. Do not be mislead by the name "robotic". Unlike a robot in an assembly line, surgical robots are not independent. It is still the surgeon who controls every action of the surgical robot.

During a robotic-assisted procedure the same cannulas as are used in laparoscopic surgery are inserted into the abdomen. Three or four "robotic arms" are connected to the cannulas. Then highly sophisticated instruments are inserted in the abdomen to perform specific tasks. The surgeon sits at a console a few feet away from the patient, and uses joystick controls to direct the movement of the arms.

Unlike conventional laparoscopic tools, robotic instruments are much more precise and can move around a wrist joint, thus resembling more accurately the human hand.

In addition, the view offered by the robotic camera is three dimensional, just like in open surgery, which can greatly aid the surgeon during precision-requiring operations.

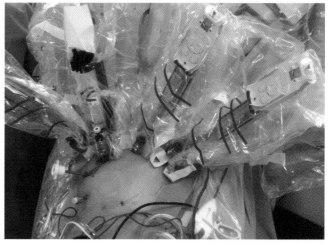

During robotic surgery instruments in sterile sleeves are manipulated by a surgeon sitting at a remote console

Robotic surgery is ideal for procedures that call for great accuracy in relatively small spaces. It is an ideal tool for prostate surgery, cardiac surgery, and, recently, rectal surgery. It is believed that the superior visualization of the tiny pelvic nerves around the rectum may help reduce sexual and bladder problems after rectal cancer surgery.

Although robotic surgery is still quite new, it is growing very rapidly and will conceivably be the most important minimally invasive technique performed throughout the world in the not too distant future.

THE NO VISIBLE SCAR OR SINGLE PORT APPROACH

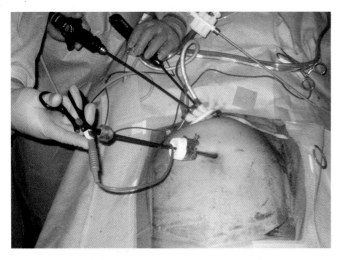

*Cosmetic results are improved by using a
single port approach*

In an effort to reduce the impact of surgery on patients even further, a number of surgeons around the world who have "mastered" laparoscopic colon surgery have developed approaches that aim to limit the incisions to only one site.

These so-called Single Port approaches offer improved cosmetic outcome and perhaps less pain. The "No Visible Scar" approach offers this same advantage while moving the scar away from the umbilicus (belly button) to the area below the pubic hair line.

SURGERY – RECTAL CANCER

Much of what we discussed in the chapter on colon cancer also applies to rectal cancer. However, there are some differences in details, since the rectum is located in a less accessible part of the body.

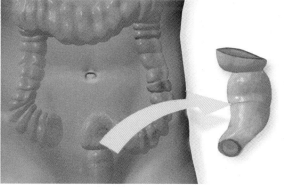

If the cancer in the rectum is nothing but a small polyp or a surface lesion, the surgeon may be able to perform a *transanal resection.* This procedure does not require an abdominal incision, since the instruments are inserted through the anus.

Surgery on larger cancers of the rectum is more challenging than surgery on cancers of the colon. The reason for this is that the rectum is located in a tightly packed area, the pelvis, and is close to the bladder, urethra, anal sphincter, nerves, and several other important structures, making access more difficult.

The main technical challenge is to remove all the cancerous tissue and achieve a cure, without damaging the nerves or the anal sphincter muscles. Damaging them may lead to *incontinence*—leakage of urine or stool.

SURGICAL OPTIONS FOR RECTAL CANCER

The choice of treatment and expected outcome depend on the exact location of the tumor within the rectum, and on the stage of the cancer. As we discussed in Chapter 3, stage is determined by:

- How deeply the tumor has invaded the wall of the rectum
- Whether the cancer has spread to the lymph nodes
- Whether the cancer has spread to other organs

CHAPTER 8

QUESTIONS TO ASK YOUR ANESTHESIOLOGIST:

- **How long will it take me to get back to normal after I have general anesthesia?**

- **Will I have a lot of pain? How can the pain be controlled?**

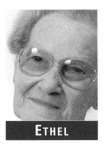

ETHEL

The tumor was too close to the anus. I had an abdominal perineal resection and a colostomy. And I've liived with a colostomy for twelve years. I don't think it slows me down any!

Stage 0 and some stage I rectal cancers can be treated with *transanal excision.* A few stage I rectal cancers, and most stage II and III rectal cancers are treated with *low anterior resection* or *abdominoperineal resection*— removal of the tumor. A generous margin of healthy tissue around the tumor has to be removed as well, to decrease the chance of leaving cancerous cells behind.

Only about five out of a hundred patients with early stage rectal cancer can be treated with this type of local therapy. More commonly, more extensive surgery is necessary. If the cancer has advanced locally, adjuvant (additional) treatment with radiation therapy and chemotherapy may be recommended. This is discussed in Chapters 9 and 10.

In some instances, such as when the cancer is large and bulky and close to the anal sphincter, or when the surgeon thinks that the anus and rectum may need to be removed, radiation therapy, with or without chemotherapy, may be given before surgery. This pre-treatment is called *neoadjuvant* therapy. The goal is to shrink the tumor enough to make it possible for the surgeon to remove the entire tumor, but preserve the anal sphincter.

Let's review the surgical procedures available for rectal cancer.

TRANSANAL EXCISION

Some early stage rectal cancers that are located close to the anus and have not spread to adjacent tissues can be removed through the anus, instead of through the abdominal wall. This procedure is called *transanal excision.* It is generally done in the operating room under general anesthesia. Your surgeon will determine whether the procedure will be done on an outpatient basis, or if you will be admitted to the hospital.

Since the abdomen is not entered and the bowel is not disturbed, transanal excision is easier on your body. But it does require a surgeon who is well-versed in this type of surgery.

An experienced colorectal cancer surgeon can often remove just the tumor and a small amount of surrounding tissue, while leaving the anus and sphincter intact. This sphincter-sparing procedure allows patients to retain bowel function and eliminates the need for a permanent colostomy.

Sphincter-sparing surgery is an option for patients with small early stage (stage I) rectal cancers that are near the anus but have not spread to the anus or the anal sphincter itself.

Before surgery you will probably have a test called endorectal ultrasound, or ERUS, to assess the extent of spread of cancer cells into adjacent tissues and lymph nodes. If there is spread, your surgeon will not perform a transanal resection, but will choose a more extensive procedure.

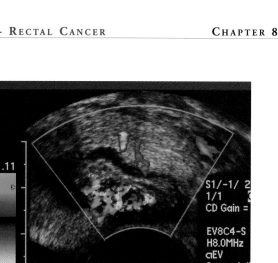

LOW ANTERIOR RESECTION, OR LAR

Low anterior resection is the surgical procedure most frequently used to deal with cancers of the rectum. This surgery is similar to a colon resection: it is performed under general anesthesia, through a single incision in the lower part of your abdominal wall. You may want to review Chapter 6 for details.

The affected part of the rectum is removed, and the end of the colon is reattached to the anus, so that feces can be passed normally.

ABDOMINOPERINEAL RESECTION, OR APR

Abdominoperineal resections use two incisions—one through the abdomen, the other through the perineum (the area between your legs, around the anus). Working through these incisions, the surgeon can remove a tumor near the bottom end of the rectum.

The surgery will involve the rectum, the anus and surrounding tissue. Because there will be no tissue left to reconstruct a functioning anus, you will have a permanent colostomy.

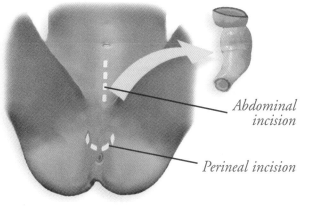

Abdominal incision

Perineal incision

APR uses two incisions to remove the cancer

Both LAR and APR procedures can be performed utilizing minimally invasive surgery (MIS) techniques described in the previous chapter.

QUESTIONS TO ASK
YOUR SURGEON:

- **What type of proce-
  dure do you think is
  best for me?**
- **What should I know
  about the possible
  complications?**
- **What is the latest
  information about
  this type of cancer
  surgery?**
- **Could I meet with
  some of the patients
  who had this proce-
  dure before?**
- **Is a colostomy
  absolutely necessary?**

Urinary function may change since the nerves that control urinary function lie in the pelvis, and might have been bruised during this extensive surgery. In certain cases, the surgeon will be able to perform a nerve sparing procedure, and preserve nerve function.

Some patients need a urinary catheter for longer than usual, or medications, or both, until normal bladder function returns. Usually, patients don't have permanent loss of urinary control (urinary incontinence).

PELVIC EXENTERATION

If the cancer has spread to nearby organs, you may need a more complex operation: a pelvic exenteration. Depending on how far the cancer has proliferated, the exenteration surgery will remove the rectum, bladder, and prostrate or uterus. A colostomy is always required for this procedure, as well as a urostomy if the bladder is removed.

RECOVERY AFTER RECTAL SURGERY

Whether you had a low anterior resection or an abdominoperineal resection, you will remain in the hospital for approximately four to seven days, and then convalesce at home for three to six weeks. If you had a pelvic exenteration, your hospital stay and home recovery may be longer.

Ask your surgeon how and when you may resume your normal activities. You may want to refer to Chapter 6, for information on how to recover faster, and improve your comfort.

Expected Results

Will the operation be successful? It is not possible to answer this question with certainty. Your expected results will depend on several so-called ***prognostic factors.***

The most important prognostic factor is the stage of the tumor—in other words, the extent of spread of the tumor into the bowel wall and beyond. Obviously, if the cancer has infiltrated the surrounding tissues, removing all of the cancerous cells might be difficult. The more extensive the surgery, the more side effects you can expect. Only your surgeon will be able to give you an assessment of what you can expect in your particular case.

Another important factor that has a bearing on the outcome is the experience and skill of the surgeon who will perform the operation. Working in a confined space, with limited visibility such as exists in the pelvic area, is best left to specialists with extensive experience in this type of procedure. Feel free to ask your surgeon about his or her particular skills, experience, and recent results.

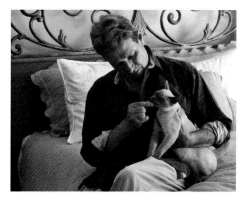

Pace yourself when resuming normal activities

COLOSTOMY

On rare occasions, depending on the size, location, and spread of the tumor, the surgeon might find that it is impossible to remove the cancerous tissue without damaging the muscles of the anal sphincter. When the anus is removed, the surgeon needs to create another pathway for the stools to exit the colon. This can be accomplished by bringing the cut end of the colon to the surface of the abdomen, through the skin, generally on the side of your abdomen.

The new opening that is created is called a *stoma*, from the Greek word mouth; since the stoma is made from the colon, it is known as a *colostomy*. The stoma will be pink and moist with a good blood supply. Since that portion of the intestinal wall has few nerve endings, you will not feel pain, light pressure, or any sensation of heat or cold within your stoma.

After surgery, a disposable, odor-proof, plastic colostomy pouch will be applied to the skin around your stoma to collect the exiting stool. Your nurse will show you how to change the pouch.

On first thought, a colostomy may sound like a major inconvenience. In fact, most patients find that having a colostomy does not prevent them from pursuing all of their previous activities. You should be able to return to work, engage in intimate or sexual contact, travel, and participate in most sports.

QUESTIONS TO ASK
YOUR SURGEON:

- **Should I talk to a colostomy nurse before the procedure?**

- **What kind of limitations should I expect regarding my sexual activities?**

- **Will my insurance pay for colostomy supplies if I need them?**

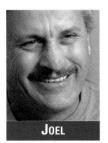

JOEL

Before my surgery, when I was emotionally feeling the lowest, the local ostomy chapter sent a visitor to see me. He was about the same age. He comes bouncing into the room, in athletic clothes, the picture of health, and he said "I've got a colostomy just like you will have." And that really, really helped.

One of the best confidence-building suggestions I can make is that you ask your surgeon to put you in touch with other men and women who have been living with a colostomy, to hear about their experiences with this device.

Another suggestion is to be sure to get a second opinion from an expert rectal surgeon as to whether you do indeed need a colostomy.

Diet

Foods that affected your bowels before surgery will continue to do so after a colostomy. Eat smaller portions of gas-forming foods, and eat slowly, making sure that the food is broken down in to the smallest pieces possible before you swallow it. To decrease gas, avoid drinking through a straw, chewing gum, and talking while eating. If odor becomes a problem, take measures to control odor by emptying the pouch at regular intervals, using pouches with charcoal filters, good hygiene, oral deodorizing agents, pouch deodorants, room spray, and odor-proof pouches.

If you are having particular problems that you think are related to your diet, speak to a dietitian or to an enterostomal therapist. They will help you select or eliminate foods that may be causing your problems, and help you manage your stoma better.

Irrigation

Your nurse will be able to give you specific instructions on how to perform a colostomy irrigation. For this procedure you will put water into the colon for the purpose of emptying the bowel contents at the same time each day. The goal of irrigation is to help the colon to develop some degree of regularity. This should allow you to remain free of drainage for 24 to 48 hours.

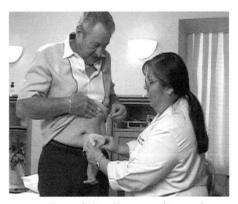

Plastic bag adheres to skin and collects feces from the colostomy

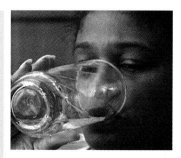

Food Considerations with a Colostomy

Gas-forming foods: broccoli, cabbage, cauliflower, corn, cucumbers, dairy products, dried beans, mushrooms, onions, peas, radishes, spinach, string beans, sweet potatoes, yams, and yeast; beer and carbonated beverages are also gas-forming.

Odor-forming foods: asparagus, beans, broccoli, Brussels sprouts, cabbage, cauliflower, eggs, fish, garlic, onions, some spices, peas, and turnips.

Odor decreasing foods: tomato juice, yogurt, buttermilk, orange juice, parsley, and spearmint.

Stool-thickening foods: bananas, rice, bread, potatoes, creamy peanut butter, applesauce, cheese, tapioca, yogurt, pasta, pretzels, marshmallows.

Stool-loosening foods: string beans, chocolate, raw fruits, raw vegetables, leafy green vegetables (e.g., lettuce, broccoli, spinach), fried foods, greasy foods, prune or grape juice, highly spiced foods.

SEXUAL SIDE EFFECTS OF RECTAL SURGERY

One issue that is sometimes overlooked is the impact of colorectal cancer treatment on your sexual life. This oversight is understandable, since when you are facing a cancer diagnosis and your life is at stake, sexuality may not be on the top of your list.

The stress of treatment, the toll taken by surgery, the side effects of chemotherapy, can all contribute to low energy levels, and loss of sexual interest. Usually after the side effects of treatment abate, you will be able to return to the same level of sexual activity as you enjoyed before surgery. But there may be physical reasons for sexual problems that may not resolve with time.

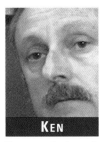

KEN

Because of where they had to operate there was a 30% chance that I would be impotent. And that prospect was devastating. After weathering the diagnosis of cancer and being told I was going to have a colostomy, then to be told that I might be impotent… But the good Lord was smiling on me because when they took out the catheter… I found out that I was not impotent.

One of the reasons is the fact that surgery on the rectum often damages the nerves that are involved in sexual function.

Men who have an AP resection may have "dry" orgasms following surgery, because of damage to the nerves that control ejaculation. Sometimes the surgery causes retrograde ejaculation, which means the semen goes backward into the bladder. AP resection should not stop your erections or ability to reach orgasm, but your pleasure at orgasm may be less intense.

Women who have an AP resection may expect to develop vaginal dryness, and may experience painful intercourse (dyspareunia) particularly if the posterior part of the vagina was surgically removed during the procedure.

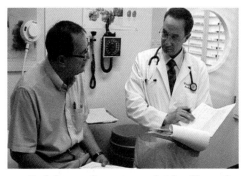

Feel free to discuss sexual side effects of surgery with your physician or nurse

Try to overcome any inhibitions you might have, and bring up the topic of possible sexual side effects when you discuss your upcoming surgery with your physician. Being prepared for the worst can only lead to a pleasant surprise. Do discuss any sexual side effects that you might develop after surgery. Your physician or nurse can offer many suggestions that you may find helpful.

CHAPTER 9

CHEMOTHERAPY

Chemotherapy is the use of drugs called cytotoxic (cell-killing) drugs that either kill cancer cells or prevent them from dividing. It is used as an adjuvant therapy (in other words, additional therapy) in combination with surgery in certain cases of colorectal cancer. After the cancer is removed surgically, your physician may recommend adjuvant treatment with chemotherapy drugs to destroy any cells that may have remained in the surgical area or spread to other parts of the body.

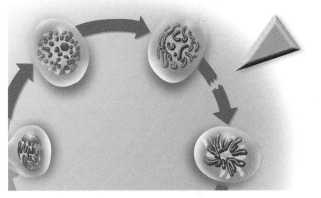

Sometimes chemotherapy is used before surgery to shrink a tumor, and improve the results of surgery. In this case it is called neoadjuvant therapy.

Chemotherapy is given intravenously or in pill form. In either case, the drugs spread throughout the body and attack cancer cells wherever they might be. For this, chemotherapy is called a systemic treatment, unlike radiation therapy and surgery, which are considered local treatments.

DO I NEED CHEMOTHERAPY?

Many patients are reluctant to face chemotherapy, because they carry the old misconception that chemotherapy is something that makes you deathly ill, or makes your hair fall out.

Much has changed in recent years. Today there are very effective drugs that can greatly reduce—and sometimes eliminate—the side effects of

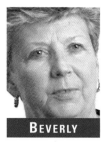

BEVERLY

Somehow taking chemo in pill form, Xeloda, gave me a feeling of being more in control… My doctor could taper the dose to make sure my blood cells where not too low. With the IV, dose goes in, they can't take it out, you know…

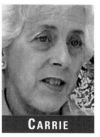

CARRIE

You hear horror stories. "The cancer won't kill you. The chemo will." But it's not true. If you can stand a little vomiting and diarrhea…It all works out ok.

chemotherapy, making the experience much more tolerable than it was rumored to be in the past.

Do you personally need chemotherapy? It depends on the stage of your tumor.

If you have early (stage I) colorectal cancer, your physician is not likely to recommend chemotherapy. Stage I tumors have not spread, and the chances are very good that surgery will remove the entire tumor and cure the disease.

There is no agreement on whether stage II colon cancer needs to be treated with chemotherapy in addition to surgery. The decision may depend on your physician's specialty.

The use of chemotherapy in stage II colon cancer is controversial because patients with stage II cancers have an excellent chance of cure by surgery alone. There is no evidence at this time that postoperative chemotherapy helps these patients live any longer.

If you have stage II and III rectal cancer, chemotherapy is a good choice, and may be combined with radiation therapy.

If you have stage III colon cancer, your chances of cure with surgery alone are less, so chemotherapy will be used to decrease the possibility that cancer cells are left behind, and to help prevent cancer from coming back (*recurring*) after surgery.

If you have stage IV or recurrent colon cancer and are too ill to have surgery, or have chosen not to have surgery for personal reasons, chemotherapy may be your main (primary) treatment. Chemotherapy will not cure advanced-stage colon cancer, but it can relieve some symptoms and may slow cancer growth.

Your physicians will help you evaluate objectively the expected advantages and disadvantages of chemotherapy. There are tests that can assess your risk of recurrence and the potential effectiveness of chemotherapy. Be sure to ask your healthcare team about these tests.

HOW CHEMOTHERAPY WORKS

Cells go through several steps in the process of cell division. First, the genetic material (DNA) in the nucleus forms strands called chromosomes. Then the chromosomes divide into two sets, and the cell enlarges. Finally the cell splits into two identical cells, each with its own set of DNA.

Chemotherapy drugs interfere with various parts of this cycle, making it difficult for the cells to reproduce and repair themselves. Often several different drugs are used simultaneously in order to target different parts of the cycle and achieve the best result.

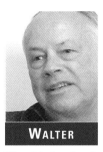

WALTER

They felt that they had resected all of the tumor, but as a precaution they put me on chemotherapy. They told me that I would lose my hair. I was already bald so no big deal. Chemotherapy was tough getting used to. In fact the morning that I would have to go in and get my shot, I would get nauseous even before I left the house.

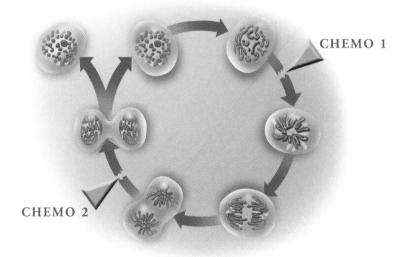

CHEMO 1

CHEMO 2

Different chemotherapy drugs block different parts
of the cell duplication cycle, making treatment more effective

HOW CHEMOTHERAPY IS GIVEN

Some chemotherapy drugs come in pill form, and you take them just as you would any other pill. Others are given by injection into a vein. These injections can be given in a private doctor's office, in a hospital, or in a cancer center.

QUESTIONS TO ASK
YOUR ONCOLOGIST:

- **Do I need chemotherapy? Why?**

- **What drugs do you recommend?**

- **What are the benefits and risks of chemotherapy?**

- **How will you know if the treatments are working?**

- **What side effects will I experience?**

- **Can I work or travel while I'm having chemotherapy?**

- **What other limitations can I expect?**

Intravenous chemotherapy is given in cycles. For example, a dose every two to four weeks. This allows the normal cells in your body to recover between treatments. The full course of therapy takes three to twelve months, but could be longer or shorter depending on your particular case.

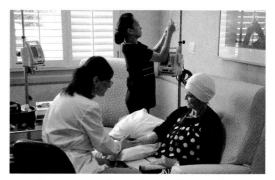

Intravenous chemotherapy is given in a medical office or at a medical center

Your experience with chemotherapy will vary depending on whether you are taking oral or intravenous chemotherapy.

The convenience of oral chemotherapy is that you will take your pills at home and probably only visit your oncologist at specific intervals to monitor your progress.

If you are on intravenous chemotherapy, you will receive the injections in an oncologist's office, or at an outpatient center. Before you receive the scheduled dose, the nurse will draw your blood, to check whether the treatment has affected the blood-producing cells in your bone marrow, or the function of your liver. If your results are too far below normal, your oncologist may decide to lower the dose, or postpone the treatment.

If your results are acceptable, the nurse will take you to the treatment area and start the IV (intravenous line) through which the drug will be injected. Then the drug will be administered. Some drugs are given as a rapid injection, others are dripped in slowly over a longer period—sometimes up to three hours. Generally you won't feel any discomfort.

SIDE EFFECTS OF CHEMOTHERAPY

Anti-cancer drugs work by preventing cells from growing and dividing. The effect is strongest on cancer cells, but normal tissues can also be affected. The most common side effects include nausea, fatigue, menopausal symptoms and hair loss. The side effects will vary with the drug used, and with your own tolerance to it.

While it is important to be prepared for possible side effects of chemotherapy, it is equally important not to assume that you will have all, many, or even a few of them. Many people go through chemotherapy without significant ill effects.

Nausea

Nausea used to be one of the most distressing side effects of many chemotherapy drugs. Today there are several effective *antiemetic* (antinausea) medications that can eliminate or decrease this problem. In addition, you may want to explore such complementary therapies (see Chapter 11) as meditation and relaxation to help relieve your discomfort.

Fatigue

High doses of chemotherapy can make you feel tired, especially on the first day after each treatment. Adjust your schedule so that you can rest if you want. Many patients find that given some flexibility they can keep a fairly normal level of activity. If you feel unable to function at a reasonable level, tell your oncologist about it. Your drug dose may be too high, and may need to be readjusted. Your physician may recommend medications to help your body rebuild red blood cells, and raise your energy level.

Neuropathy

Certain chemotherapy drugs, particularly oxaliplatin, will cause numbness in your fingers and toes called *neuropathy* of *neurotoxicity*. The side effect may be so severe that you may have difficulty holding a cup in your hands. Clinical trials now in progress will determine whether this serious side effect can be decreased by shortening treatment time.

Bone Marrow Suppression

Bone marrow cells, which produce red blood cells, white blood cells, and platelets in your blood, are particularly affected by chemotherapy, and may lose some, or all, of their function, leading to lower blood cell counts.

Red blood cells (RBC's) transport oxygen. A low red blood cell count, called anemia, will generally give you fatigue. White blood cells (WBC's) help fight infection. A normal WBC count is in the 5,000-10,000 range.

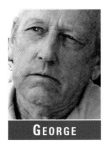

GEORGE

About three months into treatment I got bronchitis, and it took forever to get rid of it. Having smoker's lungs didn't help any, even though I stopped before surgery. I had to do antibiotics, the works. In bed at home for two weeks. They had to cut down on my next dose to let the blood cells build up till they could fight the infection.

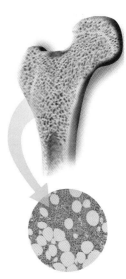

Blood cells are produced in bone marrow

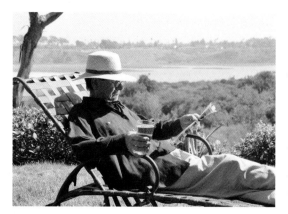

Don't over-exert yourself during cancer treatment

Platelets help the blood clot. A platelet count below 100,000 can predispose to bleeding, such as excessive bleeding from wounds, or slow bleeding into the stomach or intestine, which could appear as black stools.

Your chemotherapy dose may need to be lowered, or the treatment delayed, to avoid dangerously impairing the ability of the bone marrow to produce blood cells.

To avoid compromising the treatment by delaying or decreasing your chemotherapy, your doctor may give you medications called colony stimulating factors, such as Neulasta, to encourage your bone marrow to produce more blood cells, and protect you from complications.

Raising your white cell count will help you fight off infections. Raising your red cell count will give your blood more capacity to carry oxygen, and will improve your strength.

Infections

When your white blood cell count is low, your body may not be able to fight off infections. Most infections come from bacteria normally found on the skin, in the intestines, and in the genital tract.

Signs of Infection

- Fever over 100 degrees Fahrenheit
- Sweating and chills
- Loose bowels
- A burning feeling when you urinate
- A severe cough or sore throat
- Unusual vaginal discharge or itching
- Redness, swelling, or tenderness around a wound

Be alert to signs that you might have an infection, and report them to your doctor right away. This is especially important when your white blood cell count is low. If you have a fever, don't use aspirin, acetaminophen (Tylenol), or any other medicine to bring your temperature down without first checking with your doctor.

Other Side Effects

Some of the other side effects of chemotherapy may include mouth sores, intestinal problems, and vaginal dryness.

When chemotherapy affects the lining of the intestine, the result may be diarrhea. You can try to eat smaller portions more often, and avoid high fiber foods.

Oral Care During Cancer Treatment

- Eat foods cold or at room temperature
- Choose soft foods, such as ice cream, milkshakes, or baby food
- Avoid irritating, acidic foods, or spicy food
- Consider artificial saliva to moisten your mouth
- Drink plenty of liquids
- Suck on ice chips, popsicles, or sugarless hard candy
- Moisten dry foods with butter, margarine, gravy or sauce

If you develop sores in your mouth, be sure to contact your doctor or nurse because you may need medical treatment for the sores.

Vaginal dryness can be relieved with a variety of personal lubricant products readily available.

Some drugs may have other, even less common side effects, for example, a condition known as hand-foot syndrome, which causes redness and itching of palms and soles. Make sure your physician reviews with you the side effects that may be expected from your particular drug combination.

QUESTIONS TO ASK
YOUR DOCTOR:

- **How can I manage nausea?**
- **Will you give me medications to treat other side effects?**
- **Can I take public transportation home after treatments?**
- **Should I eat before I come for my treatments?**
- **Can I take vitamins or herbs in addition to chemotherapy?**

COMMON CHEMOTHERAPY DRUGS

The chemotherapy drugs used most often to treat colorectal cancer are 5-fluorouracil (5-FU), Xeloda (capecitabine, a pill that is activated into 5-FU in your body), leucovorin, irinotecan and oxaliplatin.

For stage III colon cancers one of the more common forms of adjuvant therapy is a regimen known as FOLFOX—a combination of oxaliplatin, 5-FU and leucovorin. Another regimen is XELOX, a combination of Xeloda and oxaliplatin. Xeloda as a single agent, or 5-FU/leucovorin without oxaliplatin can also be used.

For stage IV cancers—cancers that have metastasized to distant organs—the treatment may be FOLFOX, or a 5-FU/leucovorin, an irinotecan combination (FOLFIRI) or Xeloda—alone or in combination with other drugs.

As pharmaceutical manufacturing technologies improve, there is a tendency to replace IV medications with oral medications, which offer a number of advantages.

THE NEW GENERATION OF CANCER DRUGS

Conventional chemotherapy drugs work by killing cells, both cancerous and non-cancerous. But a new generation of anti-cancer drugs works in ways that are different, and less harmful to normal cells.

Avastin (bevacizumab)
In order to grow, tumors need oxygen and nutrients, which they get by creating their own network of blood vessels. This process is called *angiogenesis*. To start angiogenesis, the tumor produces a substance called vascular endothelial growth factor, or VEGF. Avastin works by blocking VEGF, which prevents the growth of new blood vessels, and "starves" the tumor. Studies have shown that a combination of chemotherapy and Avastin can shrink tumors and help people with metastatic colorectal cancer live longer.

Erbitux (cetuximab) and **Vectibix** (panitumumab)
These drugs belong to a class of drugs called ***monoclonal antibodies***. In

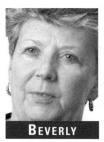

BEVERLY

I was more fearful about chemotherapy than I was about surgery. That fear was unfounded, because in pill form, the chemo wasn't that bad.

simple terms, *antibodies* are compounds produced by our own immune system in self-defense against foreign substances like bacteria, viruses or toxins. Monoclonal antibodies are manufactured in laboratories, and are designed to target a very specific portion of a foreign substance. Because of this precision, the treatment is more effective, and has fewer side effects.

These drugs work by targeting a specific protein found on the surface of cells called EGFR, or epidermal growth factor receptor. If a particular cancer is made up of cells that are rich in EGFR, Erbitux or Vectibix can be used to inhibit the growth of the tumor.

These drugs work only for tumors lacking the KRAS protein on the cell surface. Your physician will order test to verify whether you do have the protein. If you do not, you may avoid unnecessary treatment.

PERSONALIZED MEDICINE

Personalized treatment selection has been successful in breast and lung cancer. Today we have the tests necessary to develop molecular profiles that will make treatment of colorectal cancer both tumor-specific and patient-specific.

These tests are important because they can predict which patients have increased risk of side effects, or increased probability of benefiting from the treatment. This allows the oncologist to create a tailored treatment program that will be personalized to your particular case. Be sure to ask your medical team whether all necessary tests have been ordered to optimize your care.

CLINICAL TRIALS

Physicians are constantly searching for new drugs and combinations of drugs that may prove to be more effective than existing therapies. Read the *Clinical Trials* chapter, then ask your physician how you may benefit from an ongoing trial in your area. The Colon Cancer Alliance offers a service where healthcare professionals will do the research and matching for you.

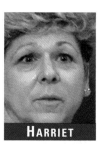

HARRIET

At least while I was in chemotherapy, I felt that I was actually doing something to kill any cancer cells that might be in my body. When I walked out of the chemo suite for the last time, there was a feeling of "Now what? Where do I go from here?"

QUESTIONS TO ASK YOUR ONCOLOGIST:

- **Do I need IV chemotherapy?**

- **Is there an alternative to IV chemotherapy that is right for me?**

- **What side effects will I have from the chemotherapy?**

NOTES

CHAPTER 10

RADIATION THERAPY

WHAT IS RADIATION THERAPY?

Radiation therapy (also called radiotherapy) uses high-energy x-rays to kill cancer cells. The treatment works by using radiation to damage the genetic material, or DNA, within the cells, making it more difficult for them to divide.

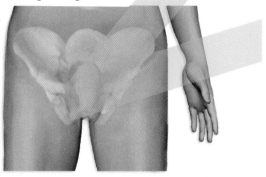

During radiation therapy both normal and cancer cells are affected, but normal cells can recover quickly, while the abnormal, rapidly dividing cancer cells, are permanently damaged. The goal is to kill any cancer cells that might remain after surgery, and to prevent cancer from coming back, or recurring.

For cancer located in the colon, the most effective treatment is surgery. Radiation therapy is used primarily for rectal cancer. It is usually given before surgery, to shrink the tumor and improve the results of the resection. Radiation therapy given before surgery is called *neoadjuvant therapy*.

Unlike chemotherapy—a systemic treatment that treats the entire body—radiation therapy is considered a *local* treatment, because it treats only the cancer area.

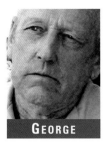

I was glad that they could add radiation to my treatments. With advanced cancer like mine, I wanted to leave no stone unturned to get better.

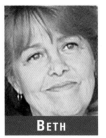

Last few days of radiation were hard. I have to admit that. I was tired. I had diarrhea. I was hurting. But I kept saying, "This too shall pass."

Your health care team may recommend radiation therapy if you have stage III cancer.

If you have stage IV cancer, or recurrent colon cancer and you are too ill to have surgery, or if you choose not to have surgery, you may receive radiation therapy alone or in combination with chemotherapy. These treatments will not cure advanced-stage colon cancer, but they can relieve some cancer symptoms and shrink tumors that are blocking the colon.

Radiation Therapy Treatment

Radiation therapy is administered at medical centers staffed by teams of professionals specializing in radiation oncology.

There are several ways to administer radiation therapy. The oldest and most common, *external beam radiation therapy*, or EBRT, uses a complex device that aims a beam of radiation at the cancer area.

Another method, *brachytherapy*, uses tiny amounts of radioactive material temporarily placed into or near the tumor.

A type of external beam radiation therapy is called *endocavitary therapy*. Instead of the beam passing through the body, a radiation-emitting device is inserted into the anus, and the rectal tumor is treated directly.

A newer radiation technique for treating colorectal cancer is called *intraoperative radiation therapy*, or IORT. This form of therapy is used for patients with extensive local spread of rectal cancer. IORT is administered after the surgeon has removed the tumor, but while the patient is still in the operating room. Since radiation is delivered directly to a specific area in the pelvis, higher-than-normal doses can be given.

EXTERNAL BEAM RADIATION THERAPY

Treatment Planning

External beam radiation therapy is used for rectal cancer and in most cases of advanced-stage colon cancer. A full course of external beam radiation therapy takes four to six weeks. The goal is to deliver the best dose to the affected area, with the least impact on the surrounding normal tissues.

This is accomplished by aiming the treatment beam at the cancer area from different angles. In this manner, the impact on healthy tissue is diminished by being spread over a large volume, while the effect on the target area, where the beams intersect, is increased. This requires an approach carefully tailored to each case.

Using a simulation unit, the radiation oncology staff will determine the best angles for the beam. Then they will outline the treatment ports— places on your body where the beam will be aimed. These ports will be marked with colored ink or by tiny tattoos. These markings will ensure that the beam is aimed accurately every treatment session.

The simulation may take several hours. The information obtained will be entered into a computer to develop your treatment plan. Sometimes a special cast will be fabricated for you to ensure consistent positioning. Once the planning is completed, the treatments can begin.

IMRT

IMRT, or intensity modulated radiation therapy, is an advanced technique that is being used more frequently in treating rectal cancer. IMRT treatment is carefully planned using sophisticated software, to plan a precise dose of radiation in three dimensions, based on a tumor's size, shape and location.

The high doses of radiation are tightly focused on the tumor, limiting exposure to much of the nearby healthy tissue.

HOW TREATMENT IS GIVEN

Radiation therapy is usually started five to seven weeks after surgery. The full course of treatment runs four to six weeks, with sessions from Monday through Friday, and rest and recovery periods during weekends.

Radiation beams are directed from several angles to reduce side effects on other organs

Typically, you will arrive at the facility at the appointed time each day. You may want to bring a friend for moral support, or an iPod or a book to help pass the time in case you have to wait.

The treatment is given in a room that has thick concrete walls and lead-lined doors, to protect those who are outside the treatment area from radiation.

The device used to deliver radiation is called a *linear accelerator.* At first the whole set up may seem complex and intimidating. But don't be alarmed. A TV monitor lets the staff keep you in sight at all times, in case you need anything.

The radiation therapist will adjust the position of the machine according to the previously determined settings, then step out of the room. During the actual exposure you must remain as still as possible. The unit will be repositioned one or two times to change the angle of the beam. Each exposure lasts only a few minutes and you won't see or feel anything.

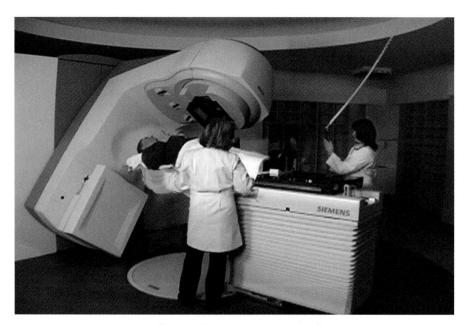

Radiation is delivered by a linear accelerator

Daily trips to the radiation therapy facility may be disruptive to your schedule. If you have to miss a day or two, discuss the situation with your doctor or nurse. You can make up the days at the end, but the efficiency of the treatment depends on having as few delays as possible.

SIDE EFFECTS OF EXTERNAL BEAM RADIATION THERAPY

Radiation therapy is a safe, proven treatment, but it does have a few unwanted side effects. Most of them are due to the fact that the radiation beam affects normal tissues around the tumor area—most importantly, the large and small bowel, and the bladder. So the most common side effects include diarrhea, nausea, vomiting, and bladder irritation. You might also experience fatigue and skin changes in the area where the beam impacts the skin on your abdomen. The side effects vary from patient to patient and according to the exact location of the radiation.

Fatigue

Fatigue is often due to stress related to your illness, daily trips for treatment, and the effects of radiation on normal cells. Most people begin to feel tired after a few weeks of radiation therapy. You can help yourself by not trying to do too much. If you feel tired, limit your activities, use your leisure time in a restful way, and try to get more sleep at night.

If you continue working a full-time job while undergoing radiation therapy, talk with your employer about adjusting your work schedule, or try working at home for a period of time.

Skin Changes

The energy waves used in radiation therapy have an effect on the skin that resembles the effect of intense sunlight. Some skin irritation and redness, similar to a sunburn, may develop by the third or fourth week of treatment. Don't rub or scratch the affected area. Use mild soap, being careful not to wash off port markings, if you have any. Wear soft clothing, preferably cotton, and protect the treated area from sunlight. Advise your doctor or nurse at once if your skin cracks or blisters, so that they can instruct you on proper care.

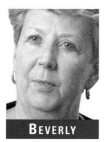

BEVERLY

The treatments were easy. But after a while I started having diarrhea. They told me it was because the colon lining got damaged by the radiation. So now I have to really watch what I eat.

Other Side Effects

If you develop diarrhea as a result of bowel irritation by the radiation beam, ask your physician to recommend a diet that is less irritating to the bowel. Avoid spicy foods, and concentrate instead on easily digestible foods that are not excessively high on roughage.

Radiation colitis (inflammation of the colon) can become a chronic (permanent) problem for many people who receive radiation therapy to treat cancer in the abdomen. Complications of chronic radiation colitis may include some of the following:

• Deep ulcers in the lining of the colon. The ulcers may bleed, causing blood in the stools. Prolonged bleeding can lead to anemia (low red blood cell count), which can cause weakness and extreme tiredness.

• Ulcers may tunnel through the affected area into surrounding tissues such as the bladder, vagina, or skin. The anus and rectum are often involved. The tunnels, called fistulas, often become infected.

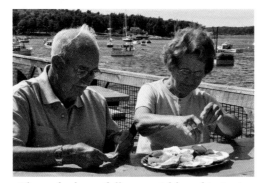
Choose foods carefully to avoid bowel irritation

• Damaged tissue in the colon may gradually be replaced with scar tissue, which cannot absorb nutrients from food, possibly leading to protein and vitamin deficiency.

• Scar tissue may cause bowel obstruction, which usually requires surgical treatment.

In men, radiation treatment to the pelvis damages the blood vessels necessary to achieve an erection, and, particularly in older men, may result in erectile dysfunction—inability to achieve an erection.

BRACHYTHERAPY

Brachytherapy is generally used for locally advanced disease. The technique utilizes seeds of radioactive material that release radiation. The seeds are placed temporarily directly into the area from where the cancer was removed, for a few days to a few weeks, depending on the desired length of the treatment.

A computer is used to determine the exact placement of the radioactive material so that the radiation can cover the entire cancer area, with the least effect on healthy tissues around the tumor.

Brachytherapy can also be used instead of surgery for elderly or sick patients who cannot endure a surgical procedure. In these cases, the radioactive material is inserted into or near the tumor.

The side effects of brachytherapy are usually less severe than those of external beam therapy, because the treatment dose is more confined. And unlike external beam therapy, brachytherapy does not require daily visits to the treatment facility.

CHEMORADIATION

To improve the success of surgery for advanced rectal cancer, physicians are using a combination of chemotherapy before surgery with radiation therapy before or after surgery. The goal of this approach is to shrink the tumor, making it possible to remove it surgically with less damage to surrounding tissues.

This therapy is becoming a standard for very large cancers that still can be removed surgically, and for locally advanced disease or tumors that cannot be removed surgically.

Preoperative chemoradiation may offer several advantages: Patients may be able to tolerate higher doses of chemotherapy before surgery, with less severe side effects. By giving chemotherapy at the earliest possible time, the metastases may be fewer or smaller, making chemotherapy more effective.

QUESTIONS TO ASK
YOUR DOCTOR:

- **Why do I need radiation therapy?**

- **How will I evaluate the effectiveness of the treatments?**

- **Which method is better for me, external beam or brachytherapy?**

- **Can I continue my usual work or exercise schedule?**

- **Can I miss a few treatments?**

- **Can I arrange to be treated elsewhere if I am traveling?**

- **What side effects, if they occur, should I report immediately?**

- **How does the cost of brachytherapy compare to cost of external beam radiation therapy?**

Other possible advantages include reducing the chance of tumor cells spreading to new locations, and improving the chance of sphincter preservation by decreasing the size of the tumor.

A possible disadvantage of using preoperative chemoradiation is that during surgery, some patients may turn out to have early-stage disease, which did not need chemoradiation.

Your doctor will discuss with you the pros and cons of chemoradiation in your particular case.

CHAPTER 11

COMPLEMENTARY AND ALTERNATIVE THERAPIES

Conventional treatments for colorectal cancer—surgery, chemotherapy and radiation therapy—are very effective in giving you the best chances for a successful outcome. These treatment methods have been extensively tested by medical experts, and have proven their capabilities.

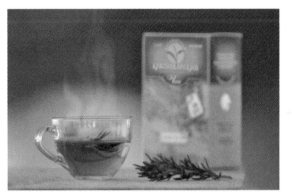

While researching your options, you may hear about other methods, such as special diets, acupuncture, new compounds, and others. Some of these methods may have a place in your treatment plan as a means to relieve some of the symptoms. Others may be harmful. It's extremely important that you understand the difference between so-called conventional or traditional medicine, and complementary or alternative therapies.

Conventional treatment is what is currently accepted by reputable healthcare providers. It is based on decades of sound medical research, and represents the best that Western medicine has to offer today.

Complementary treatments may or may not have been rigorously evaluated. They are widely and successfully used to relieve side effects of cancer treatment, and to enhance the quality of life.

Alternative therapies, by contrast, have no medically sound foundation. Instead, they may be a dangerous temptation for those who distrust traditional medical treatment.

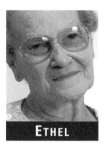

ETHEL

You need to remember that fighting cancer is a multi-faceted process. Treat it with everything that you've got. Leave no stone unturned.

QUESTIONS TO ASK

YOUR DOCTOR OR NURSE

- **What benefits can be expected from this therapy?**

- **What are the risks associated with this therapy?**

- **Do the known benefits outweigh the risks?**

- **What side effects can be expected?**

- **Will the therapy interfere with conventional treatment?**

- **Will the therapy be covered by health insurance?**

It is estimated that as much as 70% of cancer patients use some form of complementary or alternative therapy. If you decide to use either one, you should feel free to confess your decision to your physician. If you are not comfortable sharing such details with the person you have entrusted with your care, perhaps you should change providers.

In general, you can use complementary therapies while you are in remission or off chemotherapy, but during periods of active treatment you should discuss the issue with your physician.

COMPLEMENTARY THERAPIES

There is a wide variety of complementary techniques, some based on principles adopted from other specialties (for example, relaxation), from Oriental medicine (acupuncture) from Indian medicine (yoga), or even from ancient Egyptian culture (aromatherapy.)

Mind/Body Connection

Many complementary therapies are based on the principle of mind/body connection: the powerful correlation between the state of the mind and the health of the body.

Changes in the state of the nervous system, which can be caused by stress or lack of social support, can influence many of the other organ systems. For example, it has been found that people under stress are more likely to develop colds.

Anxiety, grief and fear of the unknown all seem to have a negative impact on the body. Learning how to cope with these emotions, using a wide variety of approaches—such as meditation and visualization, spiritual support, and participation in support groups—may help speed your recovery, and benefit your health.

Meditation

There is no claim that meditation cures cancer, but studies have proven that it can reduce pain, nausea and other uncomfortable side effects of cancer treatment.

Meditation and relaxation have been shown to decrease blood pressure, respiration rate, and metabolism—all of which contribute to reducing stress on our minds and bodies.

Spiritual Support

Prayer, laying on of hands, and many forms of spiritual imagery or inner dialogue have helped patients find the higher strength within themselves to cope with cancer and other illness.

Even those who have little or no connection with religion, often find themselves moved by the "spiritual emergency" of cancer.

Humor and Laughter

Laughter can stimulate your body to produce endorphins—natural chemicals that act like opiates in the brain. You might find humor and laughter emotionally healing. In addition, giving yourself time not to think about your cancer can have a wonderfully invigorating effect. Treat yourself to a comedy movie, or read a joke book. It may prove a welcome addition to your daily routine.

Acupuncture

The theory behind acupuncture is that a "vital energy" or "life force" controls the function of our organs. This life force flows along *meridian lines*. Diseases are caused by an imbalance in this flow. By inserting needles at specific points on the body, called *meridian points*, normal flow can be restored, and the disease cured.

Current research suggest that acupuncture may work by triggering the release of natural pain inhibitors. A number of western physicians have successfully used acupuncture to relieve nausea, pain or other symptoms associated with cancer.

Vitamins, minerals, antioxidants

A variety of compounds, including certain vitamins, minerals and antioxidants have been used with varying success to decrease the side effects of cancer treatment, speed recovery and improve well being. Ask your healthcare team to review the latest evidence with you.

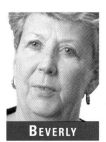

BEVERLY

I read motivational literature and practical self-hypnosis books. I took vitamins, especially C, E, and beta carotene. I rode my exercise bike almost daily. And I really found myself enjoying just plain stupid slapstick comedies…

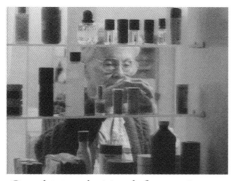

Consult your physician before starting any complementary or alternative therapy

ALTERNATIVE TREATMENTS

From time to time, a new product suddenly appears, and is promoted as a miraculous alternative to standard medical treatment. Most of the time, the claims are founded on a few poorly documented cases of alleged cures, and driven by nothing but a promoter's greed or ignorance.

It is easy to understand how a person undergoing treatment for a disease that is life threatening, may be tempted to pursue anything that guarantees a cure. Those who succumb to the temptation run the risk of disappointment, or medically disastrous results.

If you find yourself considering an unproven therapy, particularly if it is at the exclusion of a proven method, do yourself a favor: discuss your thoughts with your physician.

Tips for Spotting False Claims

• The product is advertised as a quick and effective cure-all for a wide range of ailments.

• The promoters use words like "scientific breakthrough", "miraculous cure", "exclusive product", "secret ingredient" or "ancient remedy."

• The promoter claims the government, the medical profession or research scientists have conspired to suppress the product.

• The advertisement includes undocumented cases claiming amazing results.

• The product is advertised as available from only one source, and payment is required in advance.

• The promoter promises a no-risk "money-back guarantee."

CHAPTER 12

CLINICAL TRIALS

Scientists are constantly searching for better ways of dealing with cancer. This search is done in the form of *clinical trials*. A clinical trial is an evaluation of a new way of managing cancer—with a new drug, a new procedure or a new diagnostic tool.

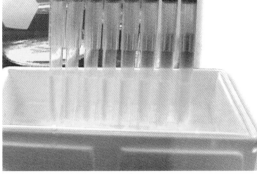

You may be reluctant to participate in what you might think is just an "experiment" with you as the "laboratory rat." Nothing could be further from the truth. Clinical trials are conducted according to very specific guidelines developed by highly trained specialists, and carried out in steps, or phases.

Phase I trials assess the safety of the treatment.

Phase II assess the effectiveness. Patients are carefully monitored for improvement and for side effects.

Phase III trials are conducted on thousands of patients in centers across the country. To reach this stage the treatment method or drug must have demonstrated that it offers potential benefits, without unacceptable risks.

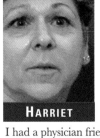

HARRIET

I had a physician friend of mine review the papers, and I also took them home, and had my husband review them too… I particularly liked that I would be carefully monitored. So I had no hesitation.

The patients are selected according to very specific criteria—age, stage of cancer, previous treatment, and so on, then divided into two groups by a random, computerized system. One group, called the *treatment group*, receives the new treatment. The other group, called the *control group*, receives whatever is considered the best suited current treatment.

Questions to Ask
Your Physician:

- **How do I know the facility doing the study is reputable?**
- **What is involved in terms of tests, treatments, and additional time commitments?**
- **What results can be reasonably expected in my particular case?**
- **How do the currently accepted treatments compare to the trial?**
- **What would be my financial commitment?**
- **Will I need to be available for follow-up testing?**

Every trial is conducted according to a *protocol*—a set of guidelines that spells out exactly what will be done and when. The trial is stopped if there are unacceptable side effects, or if it becomes obvious early on that either the new or the old treatment is definitely superior.

If the clinical trial confirms the benefits, the drug or treatment will be made available to all patients.

Participating in a Trial

If your physician does not mention trials, you may want to bring up the subject on your own.

How and where can you find a trial that is appropriate for you? Generally, you or your physician can obtain information about ongoing trials from the National Cancer Institute's hotline called PDQ.

Another excellent source is the www.ClinicalTrials.gov site. While this site is intended primarily for professionals, it offers user-friendly search features and lists over 100,000 ongoing trials. Simply enter the type of cancer you have, and the area where you live, and you will find the contact information and the status of the trial.

You may also choose to contact the Colon Cancer Alliance (CCA), which offers the service of trained professionals to do the searching for you.

If you consider a trial, the professionals conducting it will describe the details for you. If you decide to enroll, you will be asked to sign an *informed consent form*, to show that you understand the issues involved, the expected benefits, the possible side effects, your rights and responsibilities, and the possible outcome.

You will be asked to follow the schedule of treatments and tests as closely as possible, in order to make the information obtained scientifically sound.

IS A TRIAL RIGHT FOR ME?

Not every trial is suitable for your needs. There are specific advantages and disadvantages for each phase.

For example, in a Phase I trial, you are likely to be one of the first to be using the particular therapy. While being a pioneer may be unsettling, it may be an excellent opportunity to benefit from the next, yet undiscovered, treatment. Remember, CML, which eventually became the "miracle drug" was once an unproven therapy, undergoing a Phase I trial.

Phase II trials may feature more information about toxicity. They also have no control groups, which enables you to make the decision of receiving the treatment, rather than relegating the choice to a randomizing computer.

Phase III trials include much more extensive information on response and toxicity, and greater nationwide access. You may be randomized to a contol group, and slated to receive the best current care, rather the treatment being investigated, thus depriving you of the choice.

Whatever phase trial turns out to be appropriate to your case, it is an excellent opportunity to benefit from the best that medical science has to offer.

One of the main advantages of being in a clinical trial is that whether you are assigned to the treatment or the control group, you will still enjoy a higher standard of care, because trial protocols usually call for more frequent tests, more frequent visits to the hospital, and more thorough examinations.

There are few, if any, downsides. Your participation is completely optional and voluntary. You can leave the trial at any time. If you drop out, you will not be penalized in any way. And you will still be entitled to the best standard treatment available. If you stay, you will benefit from the best that medical science has to offer us today.

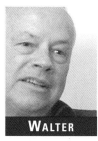

WALTER

When the doctor said, "research" I immediately thought I was going to be the lab rat. But then I looked into it, and it made sense. It was a no-lose situation. Eventually I felt very fortunate that I got to benefit from it.

NOTES

CHAPTER 13

LIFE AFTER COLORECTAL CANCER

As the treatments end and your energy and confidence return, you'll be able to move forward from the cancer experience to a new life, and you will become part of a more than a million-strong community of colorectal cancer survivors.

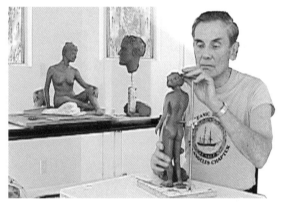

EMOTIONAL RECOVERY

A diagnosis of cancer impacts your self-esteem, your body image, your sexuality—even your outlook on survival. You probably realize that life will never be the same after such an experience. This will leave you with a sense of loss. Take time to grieve the loss. This grieving process is an important first step toward the healing of the mind.

On the bright side, the cancer experience can be a powerful incentive to reorder your priorities. To eliminate from your life the unimportant negatives and concentrate on enjoying the positives. You may decide to do something you always wanted to do—write poetry, travel, or spend more time with your grandchildren. Make a point of finding something enjoyable in every day, in every task.

Many survivors embrace the experience and become involved in a patient advocacy group. Becoming part of the survivor community and helping others can be an empowering experience.

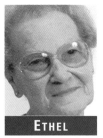

ETHEL

You know what I learned? To use my "good" china everyday. To play with my grandchildren, instead of dusting under the beds. To enjoy each day. The wake up call said: "Use your time wisely. It is not unlimited."

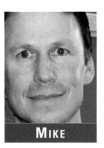

MIKE

After my recovery I wanted to help others. As firefighters we are not used to "calling 911." We are not used to asking for help. So a support group for firefighters made sense - because we already have a common bond. It's been very gratifying to create a support organization specifically for other firefighters like myself.

PHYSICAL RECOVERY

This may be a good time to adopt *healthy habits*. Good nutrition may speed your healing after surgery. A balanced diet, with proper amounts of protein, fats, carbohydrates, and vitamins will help you feel younger and stay healthier.

Physical activity will help you stay stronger and feel younger. There is also evidence that exercise can improve the immune system, and help protect you against cancer and other diseases. In addition, physical activity increases colon mobility and has a protective effect on the colon lining.

While you are working on decreasing your colon cancer risk, why not take the opportunity to adopt additional healthy habits: stop smoking, reduce or eliminate your intake of alcohol, and protect your skin against the sun.

Other lifestyle changes may help you in your personal and professional life as well: learn to practice relaxation, try meditation, and be sure to get plenty of sleep.

REGULAR FOLLOW-UP

Even after the most complete treatment, there's always a chance that cancer will recur. You are also at greater risk for a new cancer in your colon or rectum. Therefore, regular follow-up is vital. Remember, colorectal cancer can be prevented!

The follow-up could be done by your family physician, your oncologist, or your surgeon. What's important is to have a single person in charge, to ensure continuity of care.

What does follow-up involve? Your physician will discuss any unusual symptoms you might be having, perform a physical examination, and order tests. The tests may include a CEA blood test, PET, CT or MRI scans, and regular colonoscopies. Colonoscopy is the most important tool for finding evidence of possible recurring cancer, such as a new polyp. Do not neglect it! It may save your life.

RECOMMENDATIONS FOR YOUR FAMILY MEMBERS

Only about 20% of colorectal cancer is transmitted genetically, like the color of your eyes or hair. Most cases of colorectal cancer are not linked to family history.

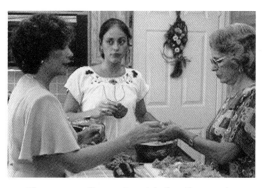

Share your diagnosis with family members

If you had colorectal cancer or polyps were found on a colonoscopy, inform your family members of your diagnosis, and suggest that they be particularly thorough in practicing early detection.

PREVENTING COLORECTAL CANCER

The most encouraging fact about colorectal cancer is that you can actually reduce your risk of ever developing it, or of having a recurrence. On the other hand, it is important to remember that even after treatement, you are not immune: you remain at risk for a new tumor.

There is some evidence, but no solid data, that certain dietary changes and physical exercise can play an important role in decreasing recurrence.

There are three major clinical trials that are expected to optimize future approach to risk reduction. One is evaluating the potential effect of *statins*, the cholesterol lowering drugs. Another is focused on NSAIDs, like Advil, and a third is studying Polyamine Synthesis Inhibitors. You may want to read the chapter on clinical trials and consult your medical team about participating in these, or similar trials.

When your treatment is complete, take advantage of the "learning moment" to adopt lifestyle practices that could improve your well-being in general, and decrease your risk of recurrence.

The most important preventive tool available is regular screening. Screening makes it possible to find and remove polyps before they have a chance to turn into cancer. Do not shortchange yourself on this potentially life-saving procedure.

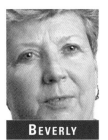

BEVERLY

The five-year check up was huge. Huge. The best news I could ever get. They said, "Well, we're not going to say you're cured, but we don't want to see you until about two years from now." That was great news.

COLORECTAL CANCER SCREENING

There are several tests that can be used, alone or in combination, to detect the early signs of colorectal cancer. You are probably already familiar with these, but your relatives may not be. Impress upon them that the best way to prevent colorectal cancer is to find it early. Some of the more common tests include:

• *Tests that detect tiny amounts of blood in the stool.*

A special test, called *fecal occult blood test* (FOBT), can detect extremely small amounts of blood, and act as a warning. The doctor will provide you with a kit to collect a stool sample that you will send to the laboratory.

The *fecal immunochemical test* (FIT) is a newer test that also detects occult blood in the stool. Some people may find it easier to use because there are no drug or dietary restrictions (vitamins or foods do not affect the FIT) and sample collection may take less effort.

FOBT and FIT may not detect a tumor that is not bleeding, so multiple stool samples should be tested.

• *Tests that use x-rays to examine the lining of the bowel.*

The colon lining can be examined with one of two x-ray procedures. One is called a *barium enema*. The colon is filled with a substance that blocks x-rays, and outlines abnormal structures like polyps.

The other is *CT colonography*, also called *virtual colonoscopy*, where a CT scan and sophisticated software yield an image almost as clear as if the colon lining were being examined visually.

The preparation or "prep" for either procedure may include a liquid diet for two days before the procedure, laxatives the night before, and an enema the morning of the exam.

The drawback to either procedure is that if something is found, you may still need to have a colonoscopy.

• *Tests that use flexible tubes that are inserted into the colon.*

The lining of the bowel can be examined directly with special flexible optical tubes equipped with a light source.

The procedure is called a ***sigmoidoscopy*** if only the last foot of the large bowel is examined. It is called a ***colonoscopy*** if the entire large bowel is checked.

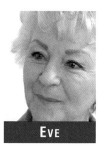

EVE

When I go for the checkup the doctor does the colonoscopy. If he finds a nodule or something, he immediately takes it out and checks it for any cancerous cells. I don't find it necessary to be put to sleep. The colonoscopy is not a terrible thing. It really is not very painful and you can have it done in ten, fifteen minutes.

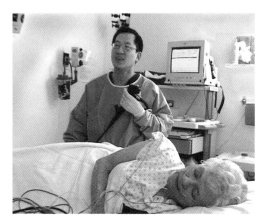

Colonoscopy is one of the most effective screening methods for colorectal cancer

Both procedures require that the bowel be as clean as possible. The bowel preparation, or "prep" may include two days of liquid diet and cleansing with laxatives, and an enema the morning of the exam. Medications may be used for sedation during the procedure. Abnormal changes can be biopsied and examined for cancer. If a polyp is found, the physician can remove it.

In the opinion of many experts, the best weapon against colorectal cancer is colonoscopy because this procedure enables a physician not only to detect a polyp if one is present, but also to remove it at the same time.

Whether you and your physician decide to use test for occult blood, x-rays, CT colonography or colonoscopy, there is one thing to remember: Any test is better than no test. Early detection is your best protection!

NOTES

CHAPTER 14

A GUIDE FOR YOUR PARTNER

If you are the spouse or life partner of someone who has just been diagnosed with colorectal cancer, now is the time to be the best companion you can be. Your spouse needs you now probably more than ever.

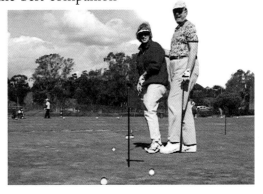

Even if yours is not a long-term relationship—perhaps you just met, or you are the patient's closest or only friend—you now have an opportunity to do something truly meaningful, something that will make a real difference in another human being's life. Consider this opportunity a gift not to be missed.

A note on the wording: to avoid long lists of possible relationships, I'll be using "partner" or "spouse" to mean you, the caregiver, whatever your special relationship may be. I'll also use he, she, her or him, randomly and interchangeably to avoid the clumsy "s/he" or "him/her."

WHAT IS COLORECTAL CANCER?

You may have heard that colorectal cancer requires a big operation, leaves you disfigured by a plastic stool-collection bag, or sends you to chemotherapy, which makes your hair fall out. And then it kills you.

Nothing could be further from the truth. Like many cancers, colorectal cancer that is diagnosed early is very treatable. And unlike most cancers, it is even preventable.

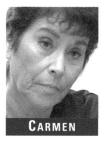

CARMEN

When I would lay there, awake all night, the most important… the only thing, really, that I wanted to hear him say is that he would be by me through this whole thing.

Begin by reviewing the appropriate chapters of this book with your partner. Understanding the disease will help you regain a feeling of control over your lives.

UNDERSTANDING YOUR FEELINGS

"I have cancer" may be the most painful words you'll ever hear from someone you love. Words that cause shock, disbelief, and confusion, and make you wonder, "Is my loved one going to die?"

Being responsible for providing both emotional and physical support is challenging. You're probably in as much pain and turmoil as your partner, but your burden may be heavier: you have to provide the support needed, as well as to deal with your own feelings.

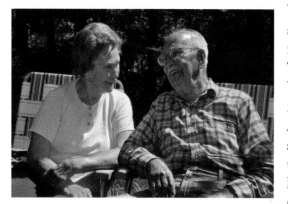

You may need to provide both emotional and physical support for your spouse

You may feel overcome by the feeling that somehow you must make it all better, and be frustrated when you find out you can't. There is no easy answer, and no shortcut. You are facing a serious problem, and it is normal to feel scared, confused, and weak. Acknowledge these feelings. You can be strong and supportive without holding everything inside. In fact, sharing your feelings honestly is the best thing you can do to strengthen the relationship.

If you find it too hard to express these feelings to your partner, you can find a support person for yourself. A friend, another family member, a religious leader, a counselor, or a support group for caregivers can help you verbalize what you are feeling, sort it all out, and work on a plan of action.

The first weeks after the diagnosis may feel like an emotional roller coaster. The swings of feelings are painful and exhausting, but they are normal. With time the emotional tidal waves fade to be mere ripples in a pool, and you find that you can deal with them.

WHAT DO I DO NOW?

One of the most constructive actions you can take is to get involved in your spouse's care. Read the general chapters in this book, then concentrate on the chapters that discuss the specific type of treatment that she will have. Learn all you can about the disease and the most current treatment options.

Get to know the *patient navigator* (sometimes called the nurse navigator) assigned to your spouse. This healthcare professional will be an invaluable companion who will help both of you during treatment and recovery.

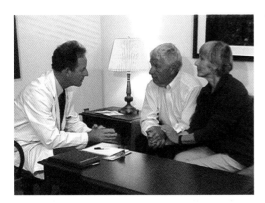

Your spouse needs your participation during visits to doctors

Accompany your spouse on visits to the healthcare specialists. Your presence will provide emotional support and a second set of ears.

Bring a list of questions you want answered. Take notes, or use a recorder. If at first you are confused, don't worry. Colorectal cancer treatment is a complex topic, and no one can grasp all the details on the first pass.

If either of you feel you need a second opinion, don't hesitate to ask for a referral, or seek one on your own. For something as important as cancer treatment, you should leave no avenue unexplored, and no reputable physician will resent your request.

A diagnosis of cancer is seldom an emergency. You and your partner have several weeks to make important treatment decisions. Don't let anyone rush you. Above all, remember that the final decisions about treatment will be your partner's. Being supportive and helpful does not mean taking over completely.

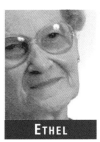

ETHEL

Even when I was thin and pale and hairless, he made me feel like a star.

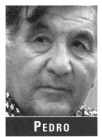

PEDRO

When I found out that Carmen had cancer, I had no family up here and my friends only had pity for me, and that was the last thing I really needed. I needed to find a place where I could sit and talk and share my fears about losing my wife. That's where joining a support group really helped.

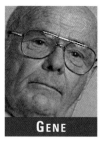

GENE

My Joannie has always been the pillar of strength for me. It was so scary to see her the sick one this time. I felt so helpless. It took some major buckling up to start to feel that it was my turn, and I had to be the strong one now. Still don't know how I did it. But I did it.

WHAT YOUR SPOUSE NEEDS FROM YOU

Emotional Support

Emotional support is perhaps the single most important factor you can contribute. Knowing that you will be there, no matter what, will help your spouse deal with the diagnosis, and tolerate the treatments.

If you find verbal communication to be difficult, and choose to hide in your job or in an outside activity, your spouse may perceive this behavior as a withdrawal of your love. Her well-being depends on your willingness to communicate openly. You don't need to make long speeches. Holding hands, sitting close, putting an arm around her, will communicate how much she means to you in ways words can't express.

Most people, especially men, are upset by tearful outbursts. But remember that tears are a healthy response. Both of you know that there is no easy fix, and to pretend otherwise only delays the grieving that must take place before healing begins.

Anger is also a normal response that needs an outlet. The patient may lash out at the closest person during such times. Despite what he says, he is not angry at you, but at his loss of control over his life. This stage will pass faster if you help direct that anger into action against the cancer.

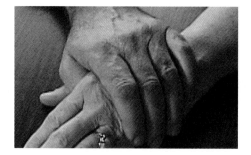

Some patients withdraw and refuse to share their feelings, rejecting your efforts at being close. This may be the most difficult reaction to deal with, and may require outside help to reestablish open communications.

There is scientific evidence that a positive mind-set can lead to an improved outcome. A supportive and upbeat attitude on your part will be contagious and is one of the best ways to help him through the weeks or months of treatment.

Sexual Intimacy

Colorectal cancer can adversely affect sexual desire and sexual function. Your spouse may need time to adjust to the effects of treatment, including possible impotency as a result of pelvic surgery. You may need time to shift your concerns away from caregiver duties and to intimate realtions. There are small things you can do to rekindle the interest. Make a date, offer a foot rub, take a shower together, watch an erotic movie. Try new positions that may be more comfortable. And remember, making love need not necessarily include intercourse.

A few simple techniques that will improve communications

- Make opening statements that let your partner know you're willing to listen. Comments like, "How do you feel about...," let her know it's okay to open up on an emotional level.

- Reassure her that she has been truly understood by repeating what you heard in your own words.

- Use nonverbal (body language) techniques to convey how you feel about her. Hand holding, and looking at her when she speaks, tell her that your love and concern are real.

- Avoid judgmental comments like, "You shouldn't...," or, "Don't say that." Such statements block true communication by minimizing or invalidating the other person's feelings.

- Be careful with comments like, "Don't worry," or, "Nothing will happen." Having a positive attitude doesn't mean being unrealistic.

Help with Daily Activities

Surgery, chemotherapy, and emotional stress may lead to physical exhaustion, and your spouse may look like she needs your help even with the simplest daily activities. The difficult part may be determining how much help she really wants. Too much help may be as inappropriate as too little. The simple solution: just ask!

QUESTIONS TO ASK
YOUR DOCTOR:

- Do you have any pamphlets, videos, or DVD's about colorectal cancer that we can take home and review?

- Is there a Resource Center or patient library in the facility where you practice?

- Who would you recommend we see for a second opinion?

- Can you put us in touch with other patients you treated for this type of cancer, and with their partners?

- Will chemotherapy cause hair to fall out?

- Can we see pictures of what the surgical scar could look like?

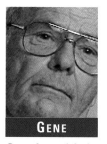

GENE

One of your jobs is to help your wife not to dwell on the bad features. Help her look forward to what tomorrow brings. Look at the scar and say, "Look how much better it looks today. Isn't that great?"

In the early stages of treatment the patient is often overcome with an excess of well-wishing friends and relatives. Your job as the spouse may be to act as the gate keeper, and delegate specific tasks to various people so everyone feels involved.

You also may be required to deal with financial or insurance issues. Be meticulous. A minor mistake in bookkeeping on your part may have serious financial consequences. Here are some things you can do to make that unpleasant task easier:

- Contact your insurance company to find out their policies on hospital admissions, second opinions, filing of claims and billing, etc.

- Keep a written record of your contacts with insurance company representatives, including names, dates, and times.

- Get to know your insurance case manager. This person will help steer you through the maze of rules, regulations and requirements.

- Write down appointment dates and doctors' names. Get a copy of all billing forms, including ones for procedures, medications, and supplies used.

- Keep copies of all bills, charges, and related forms together in one place for easy retrieval later.

- Submit claims and reports in a timely manner.

- Use certified/return-receipt-requested mail for the most important documents.

- Don't forget to keep up insurance premiums. You'll be glad you remembered this critical step later.

- Many states have a board of appeals who can help you resolve disputes. (Some contacts are listed in the Resources chapter).

MEETING YOUR OWN NEEDS

Finding Support for You

The combination of emotional stress, your regular work, and added activities around the home can take a toll on you. If you start to feel overwhelmed, make a list of tasks that need to be done daily, such as food preparation. Try to concentrate on activities that really are essential, and put off the unnecessary niceties such as making the beds. Then seek assistance from family or friends whenever you need. A simple request may be all they are waiting for to pitch in.

Fear, anxiety and stress can tire you even more than physical work. Confiding in close friends or family members can help ease the emotional burden you carry. Talking to other partners of colorectal cancer patients and participating in support groups will also help you figure out how to cope. Remember, you can't afford to exhaust yourself physically or emotionally.

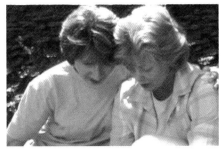

Share your feelings with a friend

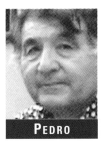

PEDRO

We thought we had it made. We were in our early 50's. We had everything we could ever want in life. Then, bang! Cancer strikes. It was all we could do, to keep plugging ahead. But our 35 years together taught us how to do it.

An excellent way to participate in your spouses recovery, give back to the community, and reenergize yourself, all at the same time, is to become involved in survivor activities. Join a patient advocacy group. Give a talk at your local library. Join a 5K walk, or attend a conference.

Suggestions for Friends Who Want to Help

- Stop by and bring a newspaper
- Bring the mail or other materials from the office
- Help redecorate a room
- Organize a getaway weekend for both of you
- Drop by and watch a favorite TV program
- Drive to a chemotherapy session
- Invite the whole family out for a meal

NOTES

Resources

American Cancer Society (ACS)
1599 Clifton Road, NE
Atlanta, Georgia 30329
1-800-ACS-2345 (227-2345)
www.cancer.org

Not-for-profit organization providing a variety of prevention and early-detection programs, as well as cancer information and support to patients, their families, and the general public. Twenty-four-hour hotline in English and Spanish.

American College of Gastroenterology (ACG)
4900B South 31st Street
Arlington, Virginia 22206
703-820-7400
www.acg.gi.org

Organization providing education on gastrointestinal illness and health to health professionals and the public.

American College of Surgeons (ACS)
633 Saint Clair Street
Chicago, Illinois 60611
312-202-5000
www.facs.org

A physician organization dedicated to improving the care of the surgical patient and to safeguarding standards of care in an optimal and ethical practice environment.

American Society of Clinical Oncology
1900 Duke Street, Suite 200
Alexandria, Virginia 22314
703-299-0150
www.asco.org

The society is a leading cancer organization for scientific and educational exchange and is an active advocate on behalf of cancer patients and their healthcare providers.

American Society of Colon & Rectal Surgeons
85 West Algonquin Rd., Suite 550
Arlington Heights, IL 60005
847-290-9184
www.fascrs.org

An association dedicated to assuring high quality of patient care, and the advancement of knowledge in this field. Offers information about surgeons to patients.

Cancer Care, Inc.
275 Seventh Avenue
New York, New York 10036
212-302-2400
www.cancercare.org

Free counseling, support groups, education and information, and referrals for people with cancer and their families to help them cope with the psychological, social, and financial consequences of cancer. Offers in-person, online, and telephone support groups.

Centers for Disease Control and
Prevention (CDC)
4770 Buford Highway, NE
MS K64
Atlanta, Georgia 30341
1-888-842-6355
www.cdc.gov/cancer
cancerinfo@cdc.gov

Government organization that develops health communication campaigns, provides cancer prevention educational materials, and recommends priorities for health promotion, health education, and cancer risk reduction for both health professionals and the public.

ClinicalTrials.gov
U.S. National Institutes of Health
www.ClinicalTrials.gov

This site is a registry and results database of clinical trials in the United States and around the world. It gives you information about a trial's purpose, who may participate, locations, and phone numbers for more details.

Colon Cancer Alliance
1025 Vermont Avenue, Suite 1066
Washington, DC 20005
www.ccalliance.org
1-877-422-2030

The Colon Cancer Alliance is the oldest and largest national patient advocacy organization whose mission is to inform, prevent, and support. The CCA offers information and support from the first-hand experience of survivors and others whose lives have been touched by this disease.

Firefighter Cancer Support Network, Inc.
Mike Dubron, President and Program Director
818-890-5755
www.firefightercancersupport.org

A support organization, started in California but rapidly growing, designed to help firefighters deal with cancer issues.

Kids Konnected
26071 Merit Circle Suite 103
Laguna Hills, CA 92653
Phone: (949) 582-5443
Toll Free: 800.899.2866
www.kidskonnected.org

Provides understanding and support to children who have a parent with cancer.

National Cancer Institute (NCI)
Cancer Information Service (CIS)
9000 Rockville Pike
Bethesda, Maryland 20848
1-800-4-CANCER (422-6237)
www.cancer.gov

The NCI offers a number of cancer programs and services, including the CIS. CIS offers trained cancer staff members who can explain medical terms and issues and provide written materials on many different cancer topics.

Oncolink
Abramson Cancer Center
of the University of Pennsylvania
3400 Spruce Street - 2 Donner
Philadelphia, PA 19104-4283
www.oncolink.com

One of the most respected cancer internet resources, with comprehensive information from leading experts clearly presented.

Oncology Nursing Society
125 Enterprise Drive
Pittsburgh, Pennsylvania 15275
www.ons.org

Professional organization of registered nurses. Provides information on research, position statements, and resource areas, such as those on cancer-related fatigue and chemotherapy-related nausea and vomiting.

United Ostomy Association
19772 MacArthur Boulevard, Suite 200
Irvine, California 92612
1-800-826-0826
714-660-8624
www.uoa.org

Provides education, information, support, and advocacy for those who have or will have a colostomy.

The Cancer Support Community
National Office
1050 17th St NW
Washington, DC 20036
Phone: (202) 659-9709
www.cancersupportcommunity.org

Provides support groups, educational programs, stress management, exercise classes, and social activities at no cost for people with cancer and their families. There are branches in many states.

GLOSSARY

Abdomen
Mid-portion of the human body, often misnamed "stomach." The abdomen contains the stomach, intestines, liver, and a variety of other organs.

Abdominoperineal resection (APR)
Surgery utilizing two incisions (abdomen and perineum) to remove cancer located in the lower part of the rectum.

Adenocarcinoma
A cancerous tumor consisting of cells lining the inner surface of the colon or rectum.

Adenomatous polyp
A flat or mushroom-shaped growth on the inside lining of the colon or rectum. Adenomatous polyps may develop into cancer.

Adjuvant therapy
A treatment that is used in addition (as an adjunct) to the main treatment. For example, chemotherapy after surgery.

Alternative therapy
A treatment that is considered unconventional and has no scientifically proven benefit.

Anastomosis
The site where two hollow structures are surgically joined. For example, after removal of a part of the colon that is malignant, the ends of the colon are rejoined in an anastomosis.

Antioxidants
Compounds found mainly in foods that protect the body against damage by molecules known as free radicals.

Benign
Not cancerous.

Biopsy
Removal of tissues or cells from the body for microscopic examination.

Carcinoma in situ
The earliest stage of cancer in which the tumor is confined to the most superficial site where it started.

Chemotherapy
A cancer treatment that uses cytotoxic drugs, given either intravenously or orally, to destroy cancerous cells.

Clinical trials
Studies that compare a standard procedure or treatment with a newly developed procedure or treatment.

Colectomy
The surgical removal of all or part of the colon.

Colonoscopy
An examination of the colon using a long flexible scope to look for polyps, cancer, or other diseases.

Colostomy
A surgically-created opening (stoma) from the colon onto the skin of the abdomen so that stool can be eliminated, bypassing the rest of the colon and rectum. The opening is covered by a bag to collect the fecal matter.

Combination chemotherapy
The use of two or more drugs to treat cancer.

Complementary therapy
Therapies that are used in addition to standard treatments. The goal of complementary therapies is to relieve side effects of treatment and enhance a patient's sense of well-being.

Computerized tomography (CT or CAT scan)
An imaging procedure that combines x-rays with a computer to produce detailed pictures of the organs.

Digital rectal examination
An exam in which a doctor inserts a gloved lubricated finger into the rectum and probes for abnormalities.

Dukes-Kirklin
A system used for staging colorectal cancer that describes the extent of the disease in a patient by letter designation (A,B,C or D).

Endocavitary radiation therapy
A form of radiation therapy for treating cancer in which the radiation beam is introduced through the anus into the rectum.

External beam radiation
A procedure in which radiation is focused from a source (linear accelerator) outside the body on the area where the cancer is located.

Familial adenomatous polypsis (FAP)
A heredity condition that will result in colorectal cancer if preventative surgery is not done.

Fecal occult blood test (FOBT)
A screening test for colon or rectal cancer that detects microscopic (occult) blood in feces.

Gastroenterology
A specialty that focuses on treating diseases of the digestive system.

Gene
A segment of DNA that holds information on hereditary traits, as well as susceptibility to certain diseases.

Infusion
Slow and/or prolonged delivery of a drug or fluids.

Intravenous (IV)
Injected into a vein.

Laparoscopy
A less invasive surgical procedure in which the surgeon operates using long slender tubes inserted through very small incisions.

Low anterior resection (LAR)
Surgery through an incision in the lower abdomen. Used to remove cancers near the upper part of the rectum.

Lymph nodes
Small bean-shaped organs that filter out germs and abnormal cells. They are interconnected by lymph ducts.

Magnetic resonance imaging (MRI)
An imaging method that combines magnetic fields, radio waves, and a computer to produce a detailed cross-sectional picture of the inside of the body.

Malignant
Cancerous.

Margin
The edge of removed tissue. A negative, or clear, margin means that there were no cancer cells near the area from which the tissue was removed. A positive surgical margin (one that has cancer cells) is a sign that some cancer may have been left in the body.

Metastasis
The spread of cancer cells from the primary (original) site to other sites in the body.

Minimally Invasive Surgery
A surgical procedure using only small incisions and special tools to access the surgical site.

Neoadjuvant therapy
Treatment that is administered prior to the primary treatment. E.g. radiation may be a neoadjuvant therapy for rectal cancer.

Oncology
A subspecialty of internal medicine that employs chemotherapy, as well as nonradiation and nonsurgical treatments, to treat cancer.

Palliative therapy
Treatment to relieve the symptoms caused by cancer and help people live more comfortably. Palliative therapy is generally not considered to be curative therapy.

Pelvis
The lower portion of the torso, below the abdomen, between the pelvic bones. It contains various organs including rectum, bladder, prostate or uterus, urethra, and pelvic nerves.

Perineum
The area where the thighs come together, containing the scrotum and anus.

Polyp
A flat or mushroom-shaped growth on the lining of the colon.

Polypectomy
Removal of a polyp. This is usually performed during a colonoscopy.

Prognosis
A prediction of the likely outcome of a disease or chance of survival in a particular patient.

Radiation oncology
A specialty that uses various forms of radiation to treat cancer.

Radiation therapy
A treatment that uses high doses of radiation to treat or control cancer.

Recurrence
Cancer that has returned after treatment. Local recurrence means that it has returned to the original site. Regional recurrence means that it has returned to the lymph nodes or to tissues near the original site. Distant recurrence is the term used to describe cancer that has metastasized, or spread, to other organs or tissues.

Resection
Surgery that removes part, or all of an organ or other structure.

Robotic surgery
A surgical procedure involving a robotic device and special instruments, controlled by the surgeon from an adjacent console.

Sigmoidoscopy
A test utilizing a flexible tube and camera that enables a doctor to view the lower third of the colon and rectum.

Stage
A classification of the extent of the cancer.

Surgical oncology
A surgical subspecialty that focuses on treating cancer surgically.

TNM system
A staging system for cancer based on three key pieces of information: T, size of tumor, N, cancer spread to nearby nodes, and M, cancer metastasis to other organs.

Tumor
An abnormal growth of cells that can be benign or malignant.

Ultrasound
A painless, noninvasive imaging method that uses high-frequency sound waves to locate and measure tumors and other abnormal growths in the body.

LIBRARY

American Cancer Society's
Complete Guide to Colorectal Cancer

Written by Bernard Levin, Terri B. Ades and Durado Brooks

American Cancer Society Press, 2005

An excellent, comprehensive book with detailed discussions about diagnosis, treatment and recovery.

Colon and Rectal Cancer: A Patient's Guide to Treatment

Written by Paul Ruggieri, MD

Addicus Books, 2001

Basic information covers the standard areas of colon and rectal cancer care. Concludes with helpful chapters on prevention and early detection.

The Colon Cancer Survivors' Guide:
Live Stronger, Longer

Written by Curtis Pesman

Tatra Press, 2005

The Colon Cancer Survivors' Guide is designed to help survivors as well as their families and friends put colon cancer in its place and move forward.

Living With Colon Cancer: Beating the Odds

Written by Eliza Wood
Foreword by David Spiegel MD

Prometheus Books, 2005

This helpful and inspiring book provides a wealth of practical information and emotional support about colon cancer. The author gives fellow patients and their families hope that they too can triumph over this serious disease.

Oncolink Patient Guide: Colorectal Cancer

Written by James M. Metz and Margaret K. Hampshire

Elsevier Saunders, 2005

This book will provide you with information about various treatment options available: surgery, chemotherapy, radiation therapy, complementary therapies that comes from one of the world's leading cancer internet resources—Oncolink.

Positive Options for Colorectal Cancer: Self-Help and Treatment

Written by Carol Ann Larson and Kathleen Ogle

Hunter House, 2004

Emphasizes that colorectal cancer is a preventable disease. Includes positive stories about life after cancer by twelve survivors.

Survivor Tales: Reflections on a Colorectal Cancer Journey - video

Produced by Kathy McDonald Jones

All Season Productions, 2002

An exceptionally well produced video that offers candid glimpses into the experiences of several men and women on their colorectal cancer journey.

Understanding Colon Cancer

Written by A. Richard Adrouny, M.D.

University Press of Mississippi, 2002

Describes the anatomy and physiology of the colon. Makes clear the stages of the disease and how they affect the prognosis. Outlines various surgical procedures, their results, and possible complications.

What To Do If You Get Colon Cancer: A Specialist Helps You Take Charge and Make Informed Choices

Written by Paul Miskovitz, MD and Marian Betancourt

Wiley, 1997

You'll learn how colon cancer develops, what to expect from diagnostic tests, and how to choose the best doctors and treatment centers. Includes tips on resuming a healthy lifestyle.

What Your Doctor May Not Tell You About Colorectal Cancer: New Tests, New Treatments, New Hope

Written by Mark Bennett Pochapin

Warner Books, 2005

Provides an easy-to-follow guide to surgery and treatment options, clinical trials and recent advances in research. Champions colonoscopy screenings. A good resource for those who want to prevent, or are currently confronting, the disease.

QUESTIONS TO ASK YOUR HEALTHCARE PROVIDERS

This section contains questions gathered from the book. They are broken down by chapters with space for your own notes. Feel free to tear out or cut out these pages, and use them as reminders of what you want to discuss.

CHAPTER 1: FACING COLORECTAL CANCER

QUESTIONS TO ASK YOUR DOCTOR:

Can I bring members of my family, or a friend, to talk to you directly?

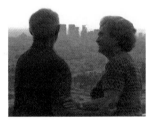

What should I tell my loved ones about my condition?

Can you refer me to a counselor or to a support group specializing in colorectal cancer?

Is there a multidisciplinary colorectal cancer team in the facility where you practice?

Could you give me the names of specialists I should see?

How about another set of names so I can choose the specialist(s) I like best?

Tell me about your, or your colleagues' experience in dealing with colorectal cancer.

Could you forward my chart, test results, and my biopsy slides to the doctor who is going to give me a second opinion?

Can you give me the name of a colorectal cancer expert who can give me a second opinion?

Chapter 5: Surgery - Polypectomy and Local Excision

Questions to Ask Your Anesthesiologist:

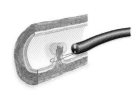

Will you give me something to help me relax before the procedure?

How long will it take me to get back to normal after the sedation?

What are the side effects of sedation?

How much pain should I expect after the procedure?

Questions to Ask Your Doctor:

How long before I can go back to my regular work or leisure activities?

What follow-up visits do you recommend?

Will I have trouble with bowel movements?

Are there any diet restrictions?

NOTES

CHAPTER 6: SURGERY - OPEN COLON RESECTION

QUESTIONS TO ASK YOUR ANESTHESIOLOGIST:

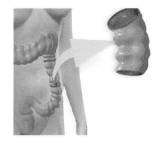

How long will it take me to get back to normal after general anesthesia?

Will you give me something to control the pain after surgery?

QUESTIONS TO ASK YOUR SURGEON:

How much colon will be removed?

How will the colectomy affect my eating?

Where, and how big, will the scar be?

How much pain should I expect in the first days after the procedure?

Do I qualify for Minimally Invasive Surgery?

How long before I can go back to my regular work or leisure activities?

Will there be any long term effects?

Will you be sending tissues for molecular testing?

NOTES

Chapter 7: Surgery - Minimally Invasive

Questions to Ask Your Anesthesiologist:

How long will it take me to get back to normal after general anesthesia?

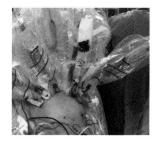

Will you give me something to control the pain after surgery?

Questions to Ask Your Surgeon:

Review the questions in Chapter 6 and 8. Some of them may apply to Minimally Invasive Surgery also.

How many Minimally Invasive Surgery procedures have you performed?

What benefits can I expect in my particular case?

Where, and how big, will the scars be?

How much pain should I expect in the first days after the procedure?

Do I qualify for Minimally Invasive Surgery?

How long before I can go back to my regular work or leisure activities?

Will you be sending tissues for molecular testing?

NOTES

CHAPTER 8: SURGERY - RECTAL CANCER

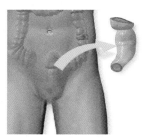

QUESTIONS TO ASK YOUR ANESTHESIOLOGIST:

How long will it take to get back to normal after general anesthesia?

QUESTIONS TO ASK YOUR SURGEON:

What type of procedure do you think is best for me?

What should I know about the possible complications?

Will I have a lot of pain? How can the pain be treated?

What is the latest information about this type of cancer surgery?

Could I meet with some of the patients who had this procedure before?

Should I talk to a colostomy nurse before the procedure?

What kind of limitations should I expect regarding my sexual activities?

Will my insurance pay for colostomy supplies if I need them?

NOTES

CHAPTER 9: SURGERY - CHEMOTHERAPY

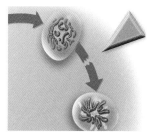

QUESTIONS TO ASK YOUR DOCTOR:

Do I need chemotherapy? Why?

What drugs do you recommend?

What are the benefits and risks of chemotherapy?

How successful is this treatment for my type of cancer?

How will you evaluate the effectiveness of the treatments?

What side effects will I experience?

Can I work and/or travel while I'm having chemotherapy?

How can I manage nausea?

Can I take public transportation home after treatments?

Can I take vitamins or herbs if I choose?

NOTES

CHAPTER 10: RADIATION THERAPY

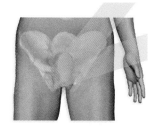

QUESTIONS TO ASK YOUR DOCTOR:

Why do I need radiation therapy?

How will I evaluate the effectiveness of the treatments?

Which method is better for me, external beam or brachytherapy?

Can I continue my usual work or exercise schedule?

Can I miss a few treatments?

Can I arrange to be treated elsewhere if I am traveling?

What side effects, if they occur, should I report immediately?

What about the different cost of brachytherapy vs. external beam?

NOTES

CHAPTER 11: COMPLEMENTARY AND ALTERNATIVE THERAPIES

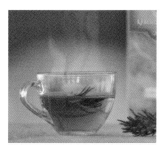

QUESTIONS TO ASK YOUR DOCTOR:

What benefits can be expected from this therapy?

What are the risks associated with this therapy?

Do the known benefits outweigh the risks?

What side effects can be expected?

Will the therapy interfere with conventional treatment?

Will the therapy be covered by health insurance?

NOTES

Chapter 12: Clinical Trials

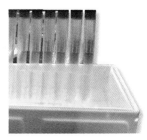

Questions to Ask Your Doctor:

How do I know the facility doing the study is reputable?

What is involved in terms of tests, treatments, and additional time commitments?

What results can be reasonably expected in my particular case?

What are the currently accepted treatments and how do they compare to the trial?

What would be my financial commitment?

Will I need to be available for follow-up testing?

NOTES

CHAPTER 13: LIFE AFTER CANCER

QUESTIONS TO ASK YOUR DOCTOR:

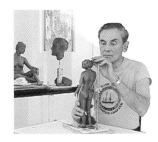

Can you suggest how I can change my habits so I can be healthier?

What factors are the greatest risks to my cancer recurring?

What is the best cancer screening schedule for me?

What should I recommend to my relatives about colorectal cancer screening?

How can I get involved so I help others who have colorectal cancer?

NOTES

Chapter 14: A Guide for Your Partner

Questions to Ask Your Doctor:

Do you have any pamphlets, videos, or DVD's about colorectal cancer that we can take home and review?

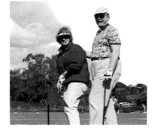

Is there a Resource Center or patient library in the facility where you practice?

Who would you recommend we see for a second opinion?

Can you put us in touch with other patients that you treated for this type of cancer, and with their partners?

Will chemotherapy cause hair to fall out?

Can we see pictures of what the surgical scar could look like?

NOTES

INDEX